//

EATERS DIGEST

The Microbiome Owner's Manual

Andy Dyer

Copyright © 2022 *Andy Dyer*
All Rights Reserved

"The individual, as he is now, is nothing else than the exaggerated expression of environment, environment being the past and the present, the inherited and the acquired."
                                                            -Jiddu Krishnamurti

Contents

Prologue — 7

Introduction: You Are Like a Tomato — 17

Part I Human Health:
Where are we and how did we get here? — 23

Chapter 1 Surrounded by Food and Starving — 25
Chapter 2 Let's Have a Caveat for Breakfast — 33
Chapter 3 We Embrace Technology — 41
Chapter 4 The Importance of Diversity — 49
Chapter 5 Biological Fixes for Biological Problems — 55
Chapter 6 Why the Rules Apply to Us — 63

Part II The Microbiome:
What is it? Why is it? — 69

Chapter 7 The Little Things in Life — 71
Chapter 8 A Brief Tour of the Human Body — 79
Chapter 9 The Microbiome: What's the flux? — 89
Chapter 10 The Microbiome: The Give and Take — 95
Chapter 11 The Human Mutualist: An Evolutionary Imperative! — 101
Chapter 12 The Human Mutualist: Guidelines for Symbionts — 109
Chapter 13 The Human Mutualist: From Costs to Benefits — 117
Chapter 14 Of BIGs and BUGs: Why Size Does Matter — 121
Chapter 15 Of BIGs and BUGs: Why The Little Things Matter — 127
Chapter 16 E = MB2 or We Need More Genes! — 135
Chapter 17 Here's The Rub: BUGS Help BIGS Stay Relevant — 143

Part III The Owner's Manual
(What you can do.) 147

Chapter 18 The Good, the Bad, and the Context is Everything 149

Chapter 19 Obligate Mutualisms: We're Inseparable Buddies 153

Chapter 20 Facultative Mutualisms: We're Just Good Friends 157

Chapter 21 Maintaining Our Balance 161

Chapter 22 How We Damage the Microbiome 165

Chapter 23 Our Chemical Romance 171

Chapter 24 Repairing the Damage and Restoring Health 177

Chapter 25 Thinking Like an Ecosystem 183

Chapter 26 Eating Like an Ecosystem 189

Chapter 27 Food Quality and Why it Matters 193

Chapter 28 Getting Your Diet in Order 197

Chapter 29 Real Food is Slow Medicine 201

Chapter 30 The Care and Feeding of Your Microbiome 205

Chapter 31 What is Food Quality? 213

Chapter 32 How Fast Should Our Food Be? 219

Chapter 33 Take Control of Your Diet (and Your Microbiome) 225

Epilogue: *A World View Based on Quality* 233

About the Author 237

Prologue

You Are Like A Tomato

The modern store-bought version of a tomato is a tasteless, uninspiring, watery, artificial imitation of a garden tomato. In stark contrast, a garden-grown tomato is the epitome of fresh food. Of all the fresh foods we eat, it's hard to come up with another example that elicits the same response from the first, the second, and the third bite. The eater's response is almost rhapsodic; no one can take a bite of a garden-fresh tomato and not comment on the flavors. Such a tomato makes so many common foods better, even special. Almost as rewarding as eating a good tomato is watching others eat one and noting their rapturous facial expressions.

So, what just happened here? Do we have a special relationship with the garden tomato? Why does the garden tomato get that response but not the store-bought tomato? Let's explore in a different way what a tomato is and what it represents, from an ecological and evolutionary point of view, and what that means to our human senses. And then I'll use the tomato to explain how and why you and I, humans, are tomatoes, perhaps more than tomatoes, but in the same problematic situation as the tomato.

To begin with, a tomato plant is really a small ecosystem nested within a much larger ecosystem. The tomato plant reaches its roots into the soil and its leaves into the air. Like all plants, it interacts with both living and non-living aspects of the external environment, and the internal biochemistry of the tomato plant is the synthesis of those interactions. The internal ecosystem of the plant works with the external ecosystem surrounding it to collaboratively produce the ultimate physical structure: the juicy, red, seed-filled tomato fruit.

The fruit is the result of the plant ecosystem interacting with the ecosystem around it. The fruit is the interaction of those two ecosystems, the product of their meeting, one nested within the other. The importance of this tightly interwoven "nestedness" is under-appreciated, and it is a key concept that seems to have been forgotten in the race toward technological improvements in agriculture over the past few decades.

What does it mean to be a tomato? The tomato plant begins life as a seed in the soil responding to different environmental cues, mostly water and temperature, that stimulate the dormant embryo to begin rapid cell division and expansion. As the seedling grows, the roots extend into the soil and begin to interact with vast numbers of bacteria, fungi, tiny nematode worms, and many other microbes and invertebrates. Many of these interactions are negative, but many are beneficial. As you would expect, positive interactions are necessary for growth, but negative interactions can also have an important influence on the normal growth and health of the plant. Some fungal interactions, such as the fungi that interact with roots (mycorrhizal fungi), provide necessary nutrients that the plant otherwise would have trouble obtaining with its own roots.

Above ground, the plant matures and produces flowers that are pollinated by bees, flies, and butterflies. The number of pollinations determines the number of seeds each fruit produces. Many small organisms roam the surfaces of the plant. Some attempt to eat the leaves and fruit while others attempt to prey on the leaf and fruit eaters.

The tomato plant not only represents a very large number of interactions with the environment, but it creates a context for a great many other interactions. Some interactions are an invariable part of the life of the plant, and others are serendipitous or chance encounters. All in all, the tomato plant is both favored by and endures these interactions.

The ultimate biological goal of the tomato plant is reproduction, that is, making as many seeds as possible to carry on the lineage. The success of the tomato plant in achieving its reproductive potential depends on the quality and quantity of the interactions between the plant and the external ecosystem. Some tomato plants will be more susceptible to the herbivores who are attempting to maximize their own reproductive potential. Others will be better able to resist and defend themselves from enemies. Some plants will respond better to the belowground microbial interactions and by doing so will gain access to larger amounts of necessary nutrients. The faster-growing plants will be more likely to receive the most sunlight and energy. Overall, the negative and beneficial outcomes of these interactions will depend considerably on the genetic makeup of each plant.

In biology, the genetic makeup of the individual organism is its *genotype*, which is the specific DNA that codes for each trait of each individual. Every gene in an individual is contained in the DNA found in every cell, but not all genes are expressed. For example, every cell in your finger contains your entire genome, every single chromosome with every single gene, yet the finger cells only use an extremely small portion of all that genetic information. The task of being a finger cell is perhaps not as complex as some other cells in the body, but all of the genes are present even if they will never be used.

All of that potential is in every cell; some is used at one time but not at another time. For example, some genes are turned off early in life but may be turned on later (e.g., the growth of body hair after puberty); some genes are turned on initially and then turned off after a period of time (e.g., fetal blood proteins are replaced by adult blood proteins after a human baby is born); and some genes are recessive (e.g., alleles that cause genetic diseases) and are best left unused and unseen. In other words, every cell in the body possesses all of the potential of the entire individual, but very little of that potential is expressed at any one location or time.

That *expression* of the genotype – what we actually see in an individual – is called the *phenotype*. This can be thought of as the expression of the genotype in a particular environment. That is to say, the environment stimulates the genotype to be expressed in different ways under different conditions. For example, in summer, an arctic fox is entirely brown but, in winter, it is completely snow white, and that pattern switches back and forth between the seasons. The fox has the genetic capacity for being either white or brown, but the cues from the environment trigger the change in coloration.

However, if the environment doesn't provide the right cues, the genotype will not express a particular phenotype. For example, the Hydrangea is a popular garden plant that produces large heads of flowers, which can range in color from white to pink to blue to purple. The particular color depends largely on the acidity (pH) of the soil, which restricts the availability of certain soil nutrients. Acidic soils cause plants to produce flowers at the blue end of the spectrum. The potential for a range of flower colors is always present in the

Hydrangea, but the environment determines what flower color will be expressed on a particular plant.

The garden tomato is just such an expression of the genotype interacting with the environment. A fully ripened, freshly picked tomato grown in an outdoor garden is an amazing taste sensation; it's a literal explosion of flavors. In contrast, a tomato grown in a greenhouse environment is an insipid pretender; it can have a granular texture, poor color, and very little taste or smell. It lacks biochemical complexity; it lacks personality.

Garden and greenhouse tomatoes can have the same appearance, but the taste and texture of each can be wildly different. They can share essentially the same genotype, but clearly not the same phenotype. How is this possible? To understand this, let's consider the purpose of the tomato fruit and its role in the evolutionary history of the tomato plant.

Every plant represents a very long record of evolutionary interactions between an organism and its environment. For almost as long as there have been flowering plants, there have been any number of insects that have attempted to eat the roots, stems, leaves, flowers, fruits, and seeds or to drink the fluids of those plants. Plants have few options in their defense against a hungry world; they can't run away and so must defend themselves where they grow. To do this, they can defend themselves with physical protections in the form of spines, bristles, hairs, and other forms of external weaponry. Or they can defend themselves with chemicals that are toxic in one way or another.

Not every plant has physical protections, but *every* wild plant possesses chemical defenses and they typically are adaptations to insects. As these defenses evolved to ward off a hungry insect world, the insects were forced to adapt to overcome the plant's defense chemicals. In turn, as insects became less susceptible to the defenses and renewed their attack, the plant was forced to adapt to produce better or different chemicals in response.

This back-and-forth process has been going on for millions of years and is the gist of my previous book, *Chasing the Red Queen*.[1] The *evolutionary arms race* is the battle between organisms in which one is typically attempting to prey on the other, the other is defending itself and, under natural conditions, neither organism ever holds the upper hand for long. Every living species of plant, for its entire

---

[1] Andy Dyer. 2014. *Chasing the Red Queen: The Evolutionary Race Between Agricultural Pests and Poisons*. Island Press.

history, has survived the threat of herbivore in its external environment and, most of the time, this was accomplished with chemicals.

As a result of this long evolutionary saga of survival, the tomato is biochemically complex. All plants produce an array of chemical compounds that are necessary for the day-to-day functions of the plant. These *primary* compounds perform all of the normal processes required for the growth and health of the plant and include, for example, DNA, proteins, sugar, and pigments.

In contrast, the defense chemicals are *secondary* compounds (metabolites) that have been derived from the primary compounds. They originated from mutations to the genes for the primary compounds that resulted in somewhat modified chemicals with new functions.

If the modified chemicals assisted the plant in defending itself in any way from herbivores, that would lead to the successful production of more seeds. If so, then that mutation would have increased survival and would have become an important part of the genotype. As an example, if a mutation to a protein molecule resulted in an unpleasant flavor, some insects might be less likely to eat the plant.

Within a single plant, we may find dozens to hundreds of secondary compounds. We assume their presence in the plant is evidence of a long and successful history of defense against plant-eating animals. These compounds can be found in every part of the plant, from the root tips to the shoot tips, and especially in the fruits and seeds. Importantly, the defense molecules in different parts of the plant will break down as the plant ages or as it passes through different life stages. The breakdown of secondary metabolites often results in smaller volatile organic molecules that are directly involved in flavor. Over 7,000 flavor-related molecules have been identified in plants.

The tomato has about 400 different volatile organic compounds, mostly from secondary metabolites, of which about 30 are also important contributors to flavor.[2] The flavor of the tomato fruit is a delicate balance of the volatile components in addition to the basic tastes, such as sweet, sour, and bitter, that may be contributed by the non-volatile components. Why are these so-called defense compounds involved in flavor and especially in what we consider good flavor?

---

[2] Stephen A. Goff and Harry J. Klee. 2006. Plant volatile compounds: sensory cues for health and nutritional value? *Science* 311:815-819. Elizabeth A. Baldwin, et al. 2000. Flavor trivia and tomato aroma. *HortScience* 35:1013-1022.

Why does there have to be a balance between toxicity and flavor? And how can a fruit be toxic now but non-toxic later? This is all part of the strategy for being a successful tomato.

Herbivores attack the tomato at every stage in life. If we consider just insects, the plant must defend itself from attacks on every part of the plant and at every growth stage. To complete its life cycle, the plant must protect all of its parts. Leaves are needed to produce sugars that are used in every aspect of growth, so leaves are vital and must be protected. Roots are needed to absorb water and nutrients from the soil to facilitate photosynthesis in the leaves, so the roots must be protected. Eventually, the plant must produce flowers, fruits, and seeds to ensure the genetic continuation to the next generation, and these structures must be defended vigorously. The defense of the leaves, roots, and stems helps the plant produce enough energy to complete the reproductive cycle, and so the defense of every part of the plant is critical.

However, the plant must also attract friends while repelling enemies, and so different parts of the plant are defended to different degrees. Flowers are chemically defended in different ways than are seeds. Flowers are the window dressing, the advertisement, that attracts pollinators, and pollinators ensure that seeds are produced. But flowers are only necessary to attract the pollinators; once pollination has been achieved, the colorful flower parts typically fade or fall away and cease to be a visual attraction.

In contrast, seeds are the offspring of the plant, the next generation, and represent a different value to the plant. After pollination and during seed development, the seeds are not colorful or obvious; they are hidden or obscured. At that point, the young fruit (containing the developing seeds) is a shifting biochemical combination of flowers and seeds. In a chemical sense, it is both defended and not defended depending on the stage of development. The attractive aspects of the flower are disappearing, and the plant shifts into a defense mode as the fruits are growing.

Until the fruit is "ripe," it is physically or chemically defended, potentially toxic to many would-be herbivores because the seeds contained inside are still developing and highly vulnerable. During this stage the fruit is not colorful or obvious.

As the seeds reach maturity, the fruit "ripens" and begins to change color. The change to a bright color that contrasts with the green of the leaves and the change in the aroma are both indicators to fruit lovers that the fruit is ready for eating. It is not only undefended but, like a flower, is being actively advertised as food. At that point, animals arrive to consume the sweet, tasty, nutritious, *and non-toxic* fruits that contain mature seeds. The fruit passes through the animals quickly and before the seeds can be digested. They are thus dispersed throughout the surrounding habitat.

Therefore, the stages of development in the tomato plant require a wide range of chemical compounds to complete the many processes leading to the ultimate goal of dispersing tomato seeds. The abundance of these compounds inside the plant goes up and down, and the numbers of compounds are surprisingly high.

The taste of the ripe tomato that we find so attractive is a combination of many chemicals, and many of them are the *last* to develop in the fruit. It is not until the fruit is fully ripened that the full complement of flavors is present. The quantities and intensities of these flavors have been fine-tuned by evolutionary selection (although also modified by plant breeders). The vitamins, proteins, amino acids, and sugars are all substances that are nutritious to animals. The wide array of volatile secondary compounds contributes to flavor, but these can be residual defensive compounds from the earlier stages of the plant or degraded primary and secondary metabolic compounds. *All of these chemicals come together to give the tomato its characteristic qualities*, but many of them are initially produced in the plant for a range of purposes.

Fast forward to today. We now grow the vast majority of the tomatoes that we eat in greenhouses, hothouses, hydroponically, and in other controlled environments.[3] Literally, all tomatoes sold in conventional grocery stores, including most heirloom tomatoes, are grown indoors in a controlled artificial setting rather than outdoors in a natural setting. They are grown in small amounts of relatively sterile soil, or often with no soil at all, and with a steady supply of nutrients from artificial fertilizers.

We have bred tomato varieties to produce enormous quantities of fruit very rapidly in a way that is analogous to breeding egg-laying chickens. The wild jungle fowl, from which chickens evolved, lays 10-15 eggs per season, while the chicken of 1920 laid 80-150 per year, and the modern chicken is expected to lay 250-300 per year. This high level of production, either in tomatoes or eggs, results in foods

---

[3] Barry Estabrook. 2011. *Tomatoland: How Modern Industrial Agriculture Destroyed Our Most Alluring Fruit.* (Andrews McMeel Publishing)

with diluted nutritional content or quality, but it's important to appreciate the many factors affecting quality.

The sterile environment of greenhouse production is a far cry from growing tomatoes in a garden. When we taste a greenhouse tomato, we should not wonder about its lack of 'tomato' flavor.[4] Instead, we should ask the much more relevant question: if the phenotype of the plant is the interaction between the environment and the genotype, then how can it be possible to achieve the natural phenotype if the environment is prevented from interacting with the genotype? *In simpler terms, how can a tomato grow up properly if it never goes outdoors?*

To grow the best tomato fruit, the tomato plant must go outdoors. It must interact with the environment to which it is adapted so that its genotype can be fully expressed. The tomato plant, like many plants, doesn't have to produce defensive compounds at all times. Many plants don't use energy for that purpose unless that effort is needed (that is, they're being attacked). Therefore, plants often defend themselves only after detecting physical damage from an herbivore.

When we grow food plants that never experience the stress of being attacked, they may not be stimulated to produce the chemicals that create the best-tasting fruit or that have the most health benefits. By analogy, a human individual can have the genetic potential to be a fast runner, but unless she forces her bones and muscles to become stronger by the stress of exercise, she will never achieve that physical potential. It is the stress of the environment that generates the optimal outcome. Greenhouse tomatoes will *never* be as delicious as garden tomatoes because their true character can only be expressed under somewhat stressful conditions, that is, conditions similar to those that caused the plant to evolve and maintain that genotype in the first place.

So, the tomato we eat should be thought of as *the physical expression of the tomato genotype when exposed to the natural environment*. The natural environment is a multi-species, multi-stress period of time in which the plant adjusts to and accommodates stress while fulfilling the evolutionary goal of successfully producing a new generation. When we eat a wonderfully tasty garden tomato, we are

---

[4] Having said that, the tomato industry has intentionally bred tomatoes (and essentially all crops) not for taste, but for productivity, uniformity of appearance, shelf life, and durability in shipping. (See *Tomatoland* by Barry Estabrook.) Some reports suggest the food industry cares little for flavor if the other marketing criteria are met. For an excellent review of changes in food quality and flavor, see Mark Schatzker's book *The Dorito Effect* (2015, Simon & Schuster).

experiencing the full expression of the plant's genetic potential with all of its vitamin, protein, and antioxidant benefits. When we eat a greenhouse tomato, we are being cheated.

These principles apply to all organisms, including humans. Unless the genetic, biochemical, and multispecies internal ecosystem of any organism is exposed to the multi-factor, multi-stress, multi-species external ecosystem in which it resides, the "tomato" of that organism cannot be produced. This is to say, the full genetic expression of each individual organism is a function of many *required* interactions with many other organisms. For tomatoes, this means being exposed to predators and experiencing stress so that the genome of the tomato is stimulated to fight back against the negative forces of the environment.

As humans, we are in the same evolutionary situation: each of us possesses an incredibly diverse world of minute organisms inside our bodies, an internal ecosystem that interacts with our genome, stimulating it to respond to stress. These interactions must take place for humans to fully express their potential. An active and strong immune system is evidence of a healthy rapport with the external environment. It is essential that our internal environment receives appropriate contributions from the external environment if we are to be physiologically healthy.

In a sense, to produce a good human "tomato," the internal environment of the human must receive good "tomatoes" from the external environment. The interactions between the internal environment and the external environment result in the proper expression of the human genome. For us to be good tomatoes, we must eat good tomatoes (in whatever form they happen to take).

Introduction

In this book, I will attempt to convince you that not only are all individual plants actually ecosystems but that humans are ecosystems, and the human ecosystem must interact appropriately with the surrounding ecosystem. We are small ecosystems nested within local ecosystems nested within the regional ecosystem.

The ecosystem of the individual is adapted to the larger external ecosystem in innumerable ways (mostly unknown), and the full potential of the individual is expressed when its healthy internal ecosystem is interacting with the surrounding external ecosystem, *which must also be healthy*. The recent research on the microbiome is clearly indicating that this is a non-negotiable criterion for a healthy life.

A second point of the book is this: organisms that are adapted to a certain environment will best express their abilities in that kind of environment. Their internal ecosystems are healthiest when they are embedded in the external ecosystems to which they are adapted. When they grow in a different environment, whether more stressful *or less stressful*, the genetic potential of the organism might not be fully realized.

In addition, if the natural environment lacks important factors or has been simplified and lacks natural complexity, this will change the relationship between internal and external ecosystems. This concept applies to all organisms, but I'll focus on humans; our ability to thrive can be either enhanced or compromised by the quality of the external environment because the external environment interacts with and determines the quality of our internal environment.

This last part should be of greater importance to us and to our world. How do we perceive our place within our ecosystems?

The concept of the individual as being separate from the external world originated with Aristotle (but amplified and extended by 18th Century philosophers and coincident with the Industrial Revolution.)

He created a worldview of the individual as an observer of nature and separate from it. This view, of course, was applied only to humans and not to the other animals. However, whether human or not, nothing could possibly be further from the truth.

At no point in our lives are we separate from our environment, and, in fact, nothing could be more dangerous for our well-being. Even before our birth, whatever our mothers ate, drank, and consumed affected our nutrition and biochemical balance. Were this not true, pregnant mothers would not be encouraged to limit their caffeine and alcohol intake, nor would prenatal health checkups be necessary. But they are. Infant health issues and mortality rates dramatically decline when pregnant women are more aware of how the outside world affects their inside world.

Humans are products of our ecosystems. We not only can't exist without our surrounding ecosystem, we wouldn't be here without it. Even more than that, we are absolutely and wholly dependent on the health of our personal ecosystem (the one we're just learning about) as well as our surrounding ecosystem (the one everyone talks about). Our internal balance is dependent on the quality of the food and water we consume because of the direct importance to our health, but that quality determines the health of our digestive systems, each of which is home to trillions of useful and mutualistic bacteria of a great many different species.

When that ecosystem is not happy, we are not happy. This is the underlying reason for the maladies suffered by many tourists visiting new countries and eating unusual (for them) food. Our internal ecosystems are adjusted to our normal diets and are temporarily unbalanced by the introduction of unfamiliar foods, particularly cuisines with different nutritional compositions. More importantly, it now appears that imbalances in our internal ecosystems may be responsible for the slew of "modern diseases"[5] that are reaching epidemic, even pandemic, proportions.

Life is the product of interactions with the environment. The interaction between our internal ecosystem and the external ecosystem is more than just the exchange of food before and after it is eaten. Yes,

---

[5] Which may include autism, obesity, diabetes, asthma, allergies, ADHD, and depression; auto-immune diseases such as lupus, rheumatoid arthritis, and psoriasis; digestive diseases such as colitis, coeliac disease/gluten sensitivity, and irritable bowel syndrome; and late onset diseases such as multiple sclerosis, Alzheimer's, Parkinson's, and ALS.

the bacteria in the gut are colonized and recolonized from outside, but the human body has far more interaction with the world than that. We have at least five senses that take information from the outside and interpret it on the inside. We breathe in the air. We drink in the water. We react to allergens. We provide a haven for bacteria, pathogens, and parasites. We are home to more bacterial cells than human cells. When the environment surrounding us doesn't help us maintain a healthy internal ecosystem, our personal health suffers. And we are simplifying and damaging our environment in many different ways. The long-term health effects of a simplified external ecosystem surrounding a simplified internal ecosystem are just beginning to be recognized, and the implications are not happy ones. In fact, the mounting evidence suggests an impending crisis.

There are a growing number of books focused on the importance of the internal ecosystem of humans, now called the *microbiome*, and the consequences for human health of disturbing that ecosystem. The microbiome is the most fascinating realm of scientific and medical research *ever,* and every person should make an attempt to educate themselves about the microbiome and its relationship with personal health.

In this book, I will not go to great lengths to discuss the latest breakthroughs concerning our understanding of the microbiome and its importance to our health.[6] Instead, this book is an attempt to take a different approach, first, by discussing how we got where we are today in terms of public health and our relationship with bacteria; second, by reviewing what the microbiome is, why we have one, and why we should care about it; and, third, how we use that information to behave in a way that strengthens our role as a walking, talking, *and healthy* ecosystem.

We'll first consider how the world has changed in the past few generations, especially our relationship with the technologies we use to modify the world we live in. For example, our single-minded focus on producing calories at a low cost has resulted in a heavy reliance on technology to produce vast quantities of food in an industrial context. This reliance on technology to solve our food *quantity* problems to

---

[6] There are already several excellent books focused on the microbiome. For starters, consider those by Alanna Collen (*10% Human*), Martin Blaser (*Missing Microbes*), Giulia Enders (*GUT*), and Ed Yong (*I Contain Multitudes*). Keep in mind all science books are out of date as soon as they are published. Think of these books as the tip of the iceberg.

feed ever-increasing human and livestock populations has come at the cost of food *quality,* which I believe has created a new set of problems.

Essentially, this is a cautionary tale: *high productivity to maintain low-cost equals low quality.* We embarked on this quest in earnest about 70 years ago with the deployment of synthetic pesticides and fertilizers. The wave of technology being applied to food production has only grown and grown – to the point that the agro-technology sector, not the wishes of the public, determines the directions we take in food production. We are now experiencing *en masse* the health consequences of decisions concerning the quality of our food that began immediately after the end of WWII.

As we attempt to understand the rapidly escalating health problems now terrorizing our societies, I will suggest that we may be asking the wrong questions. In particular, our absolute conviction that technology will solve our problems is, in my opinion, completely misplaced. Television and cable channels are inundating us with the latest and greatest drugs to alleviate modern medical problems. These are also technological solutions, and they are being offered to a public that does not understand that it is the technological solutions to food production and disease that underlie our growing medical problems. One should not take strychnine to cure cyanide poisoning.

We have to understand the role of our internal ecosystem in maintaining our health before we can manage our health. We've been aware of the microbiota of our digestive system for quite some time, but we've never considered the presence of that microbiome as something essential, as something that integrates a number of important physiological and biochemical functions in our bodies, not the least of which is our immune system. This critical emerging information must be incorporated into a more ecosystem-oriented context for us to appreciate how we should interpret and understand the complex inter-relationships between our internal and external worlds.

As we become more and more urban and sedentary and completely dependent nutritionally on what we find at the grocery stores, we must become more informed and responsible for the management of our internal ecosystems if we expect to stay healthy personally and to regain our health as a society. *In essence, we may have to re-learn what is food and what isn't food.*

As a preface, I've used the tomato as an example of the importance of the external environment to the physical and biochemical expression of the potential of the internal environment.

We need to appreciate that all species, especially humans, are fully dependent on their internal ecosystems and the internal ecosystems are fully dependent on the external ecosystem. More specifically, the *health* of our internal ecosystem is dependent on the *health* of the external ecosystem, and the health of our internal ecosystem is responsible for our health as individuals.

We not only are what we eat, but *we also are not what we don't eat*, and in some ways, that might lead to more important complications in terms of our health.

Part I

Human Health:
Where Are We And How Did We Get Here?

Chapter 1

Surrounded By Food And Starving

As we know, there are known; there are things we know we know. We also know there are known unknowns; that is to say, we know there are some things we do not know. But there are also unknown unknowns - the ones we don't know, and we don't know.

-Donald Rumsfeld, 2002

We are faced with a fundamental problem in the Modern World: What does it mean to be a healthy human? That simple question has many different angles, but it's possible the one angle that the vast majority of us ask about every waking day is: *What am I supposed to eat?*

Many of us have had a version of the following internal monologue:

"This is supposed to be the most advanced age in history, and I don't know what to eat. This 24/7 barrage of advertising is just confusing me. Can I drink my lunch, or do I have to chew it? Should I take vitamins with breakfast? Should I skip breakfast? Is it the most important meal of the day? Is a mid-morning snack bad for me? Is bread worse than a candy bar? What is good for me to eat...every day? Why is this such a hard question? I just want to go to the grocery store or the restaurant and get food that will actually make me feel better. I thought the food was supposed to make me feel good when I ate it, but most food doesn't do that. Food should keep me healthy, pep me up, fuel the fire within, and help me live a

long life. I don't think most of the food I eat does that. I think the double cheeseburger I ate last night gave me nightmares. Does everyone feel this way, or just me? Maybe I'm sick. Maybe it's me and not the food."

You're right. This is the most technologically advanced age ever. We have amazing and rapidly advancing genetic and pharmaceutical technology at our disposal. We can manipulate human genes in the embryo. We can make life-saving drugs, it seems, for every common ailment. We have vaccines for more viruses and antibiotics for more bacterial infections. We are feeding almost 8 billion people around the world. Food is plentiful and cheap. Information, energy, transportation, electronics galore, and food, food, food!

This is also the most confusing age ever. When in history did humans ever have to question the food they ate? Most of our history was focused on finding food, and perhaps trying not to be food, but our history has never been deciding if the glut of food in front of us is actually good to eat. While there have always been diet fads focused on the kinds of food that we should eat to be healthy, we have never had to worry that normal food would actually be bad for us (except when it spoiled.)

We should be the healthiest people in all of human history! So, why are we in the midst of an era where it seems we have to tread very lightly with food, or it will somehow and for some reason attack and kill us? What has changed? *Why does it seem like we're overeating and starving at the same time*?

To be honest, everything around us has changed, but at the same time, we are still the people we always were. Truly, despite the ever-changing world around us, we like to think we are a constant in that world of change. Aren't we still the same? Yes, humans in the genetic sense have not changed, but on the other hand, yes, we have changed. The how and why of that change is the point of this book, although what almost everyone really wants to know is "what do I do about it?" That answer is complicated, unfortunately, but if we understand the how and why (Part I and II), we should be able to get to "what to do" (Part III).

For starters, we keep using the word "food" to mean the meat and plants we put in our mouths to provide nutrition and benefits to our bodies. It's food; it feeds us. A one-to-one straight-line relationship.

But today, "food" may not mean what we think it means. Inconceivable, I know.

First, our food is not what it used to be, and we are the ones who did that. Unfortunately, a lot of the change to our food was rather unintentional on our part, although some of it was an indirect result of the process of intentionally changing our food for economic reasons. And then there was the fast-food part where we intentionally made our food almost bad for us. That whole thing was like a snowball rolling down a very long hill. We got that ball rolling, and it wasn't until it was HUGE that we realized we may have made a mistake. A bit late. We now live in a world where food can be good, neutral, or bad for us, and the worst part is we quite often can't tell the difference. In fact, a food can be good for one person but bad, even dangerous, for another. This is the stuff of nightmares.

Let's step back for a moment to a more basic question related to food: What is a human? Humans are in the (perhaps unfortunate) position of being at the top of the food chain. Actually, we have surpassed the food chain, we have risen above it in a sense, and we eat on any part of the food chain we want. We can manipulate the food chain to suit our gastronomic purposes, and we are not limited by predators and competitors. We can convert the world to farmland; *we are in charge of the food chain!*

Unfortunately, we aren't exactly sure what that should mean. For the past 50 years, it seems to have meant that we could eat burgers and fries or fried chicken at every meal if we so desire. And for the past 40 years, we can wash down that "meal" with corn-syrup-sweetened drinks. *And then it got worse*. It's not that the salt, fat, sugar, and lack of anything resembling an actual plant is so bad for you, but this food is like nothing our bodies ever encountered in any part of human history. It's strange and unhuman food.

Our bodies have an expectation of the food we will eat. We have an expectation that the food we eat is what it should be (and what it is advertised to be). Unfortunately, the food we eat today is not the same as the food we ate 100 years ago, or 50 years ago or even 10 years ago. Our food is changing faster than anyone is keeping up with, and we, as consumers, are receiving little, if any, information about that change. As a consequence, we are ignorant of food quality, and our bodies are becoming more and more unhappy with us because, in a very real sense, we are starving ourselves by eating modern food. It is truly possible that the food we are producing to feed ourselves and the world is endangering our future as a species.

Our bodies and our digestive systems are remarkably competent and flexible and able to handle incredible change. Human populations have shifted from hunting and gathering cultures to farming cultures to urban cultures to modern large city megalopolis cultures, and our bodies have (seemingly) handled the changes. If you understand that we invented agriculture only ~10,000 years ago, but the shift to an ultra-urban culture occurred in only the past 100 years, well, you should be both amazed and concerned.

Although our external environment changed dramatically, our internal environment seems to have handled the transitions pretty well. Yes, there were more and different diseases, but those were diseases related to viral and bacterial pathogens associated with high densities of humans. They were not due to some radical change in the human body. Nonetheless, for the past 50 years or so, we have begun seeing diseases that might be a result of changes within us.

What has REALLY changed in the past 70 years is technology (as it relates to food) and how we interact with what technology has done to our food. We appear to have reached a tipping point where we have changed too many things, and all of those changes are adding up. The problem isn't environmental toxins, but in a way, it is. It isn't food quality, but in a way, it is. The problem is a shift in our entire environment that is putting stress on the human biological system.

Our food environment tends to have a lot of toxins. Those toxins are just the way organisms (mostly plants) protect themselves from other things that want to eat them. Humans are one of those "things" that want to eat plants, so the world of plants tends to be somewhat toxic to us too. Our bodies are quite capable of handling an immense number of toxins, mostly from the plants we eat and much less so from the animals. Our liver is the center of detoxification for anything that makes it into our circulatory systems, but our digestive system handles a great deal of the load. However, in recent decades, the load of environmental toxins has greatly increased, and that's almost entirely our doing.

We now live in a chemical chaos. The chemicals include hundreds of insecticides, herbicides, household chemicals, fertilizers, antibiotics, plastics, pharmaceuticals, personal-care products, preservatives, trans-fats, vitamins, and so on. These chemicals surround us; they're in us, we consume them, we can't escape them, and they are changing both the external world and the internal human world. As far as our bodies are concerned, toxins are toxins, whether they come from our food or elsewhere. Toxins are something our bodies have to handle one way or another.

We can think of any chemical as a stress to our body because if the chemical changes our biochemistry in any way, then it is a stress the body must deal with. For the most part, our bodies are well-equipped to handle these and other stresses, but if the cumulative impact of the stresses overwhelms the body systems or changes them in any way that makes our systems less able to handle stress, then we are faced with possible chronic illnesses.

Modern life is full of stresses. There probably isn't any way around that. We have exercise, hobbies, distractions, eating, drinking, and forms of bingeing, and it's all about handling the stresses of modern life. The reason that many of us have adopted aspects of Eastern cultures, such as meditation and yoga, is that we are attempting to manage stress. Admittedly, what we probably all need is just to eat better and sleep more, but stress has a way of interfering with good intentions. And unfortunately, some of the invisible stresses in our lives may be tampering with the machinery and making sleep and weight management, and general good health all but impossible.

Stress is one of those variables that influences other variables in negative ways. If stress causes sleeplessness, it affects the body's ability to recover from one day to the next. The body is then weaker and less able to handle additional stress. One of the variables that is greatly affected is our immune system. I've taught high school and university students for 25 years, and I find myself in conversations like this one:

"Professor, I'm sorry I missed class, but I got a cold from my friend last weekend."

"From your friend? How did you do that?"

"We went to the beach last weekend, and she had a cold, and now I have it."

"What kinds of things were you doing at the beach?"

"Oh! It was a non-stop beach party for the whole weekend!"

"Just out of curiosity, how much sleep did you get last weekend?"

"Haha! MAYBE 4 hours the whole weekend!"

What my students rarely know is that the cold virus (a rhinovirus) lives in our nose and nasal cavity all the time. We carry it around with us 24/7/365, and each of us may have our own strain of it. That doesn't mean we get a cold every ten days, but it does mean that if the conditions change and our immune system is weakened for any reason, the virus may begin to grow unchecked... and we get a head cold.

What could have weakened my student's immune system? Alcohol, food, lack of sleep, and her own microbiome (as well as other microbiomes) all intersected last weekend, and her immune system was the victim. Her otherwise strong immune system usually keeps the resident cold virus at bay and she lives her life not knowing that she carries that virus and probably several others. We all do. It isn't a problem for us although we, as carriers, can certainly cause problems for other people with compromised or naïve immune systems.

Our modern life of stress is changing us in ways we don't understand. Perhaps, we don't need to fully understand. We intuitively know that being physiologically weakened in this world is not ever going to be a positive situation. We can intuitively know that if we are faced with an external world of toxins that is growing daily, then we must be physiologically strong. Our internal environment must be at its best. And the human body is a strong system that has survived some pretty incredible challenges in the past 10,000 years.

So, the big question is, "How do we do this?" One, we have to do it together, and two, let's talk about the microbiome now.

Basically, we're home to thousands of other species of life, both on us and especially in us, and this arrangement is not an accident of nature. We are their house and home. Some are transient and some are permanent; some are necessary to us and some can't live without us. The microbiome of the TV advertising world is the 10,000 (and counting) species of bacteria numbering in the trillions that live in the colon (large intestine) and feed on the undigested food material from our daily meals. It would appear that the microbiome is absolutely necessary for a healthy life although we know next to nothing about who the players are, what they do, and how they interact. In later chapters, I'll describe that in more detail, but, honestly, we don't know much. Here, I want to point out that the microbiome (somehow!) is very likely a major part of our stress-management system.

We are just beginning to understand what this means. It has become apparent that the immune system is not only influenced by the microbiome, it may be a *product* of the microbiome. The microbiome may be the reason we have a healthy and strong immune system. That is, the *healthy* microbiome may be the reason because the disturbed, simplified, or *unhealthy* microbiome can also be the root of a number of diseases that are reaching epidemic proportions in the world. And if you find this just adds unpleasant complication to an already complicated daily life, you are not alone! As if the world and life weren't complicated enough, now we have this world of bacteria in our colon that we don't understand…and its happiness is a key to our happiness?

Sorry about that, but yes. My goal here is to discuss this in a way that allows us to proceed without having to get a PhD in microbiology or biochemistry. And anyway, I also believe we don't have time for that, but we can make some informed decisions now, and we just need to go over some basic ecology and general science.

Chapter 2

Let's Have A Caveat For Breakfast

First, there is no such thing as good or bad bacteria. That might raise some eyebrows. The entirety of the advertising world will disagree with that statement, as well as a good portion of the medical world, but it's true. If you watch TV, you know that a growing number of food products like prebiotic products will "feed the good bacteria" or that "good bacteria" can be supplied by probiotic yogurts and those bacteria somehow suppress the bad bacteria. Honestly, that isn't how bacteria work.

Bacteria are tiny organisms that feed on large organic molecules by breaking them down with an array of enzymes. We do the same thing with our digestive enzymes in the small intestine. When bacteria are in a good environment, they reproduce by basically splitting in two. The more food molecules there are for bacteria, the faster they can split in two, and the more bacteria there are. One happy bacterium can produce prodigious numbers of descendants in a very short time (for example, ~60 billion in 12 hours). If there is a particular food item, the bacteria that are best at eating it will grow faster than other bacteria and basically will take over.

Bacteria (and fungi) are old. They have been trying to eat the dead material in the world for a very long time, and they are serious competitors with each other. In fact, to influence the outcome of competition with each other, they often produce toxins to discourage other species of bacteria and fungi from trying to eat their food. Many of these toxins that can kill other microbes have been given a name by humans: antibiotics (that is, they are 'anti-life'). It's likely that most, if not all, bacteria have some form of chemical defense for discouraging other microbial competitors.

When we encounter bacteria that cause disease, we consider them "bad" because they attack *us*, and we take that personally. Some bacteria get a reputation for being bad, but that can be problematic because that label is pretty general and may not always be true. For example, we get very concerned when we detect "coliform bacteria" in drinking water and swimming pools. Coliform bacteria are primarily forms of *Escherichia coli* (*E. coli*) which is a bacterium found in literally every human and mammalian gut. Yours and mine, right now.

E. coli is not usually harmful; it can break down lactose sugar from the dairy products we eat and may even be a necessary inhabitant of our large intestine for our health. However, being a bacterium, *E. coli* can reproduce fantastically fast and, being a bacterium, it generates a lot of mutations. So, while the *E. coli* I have in my colon are harmless to me, they may be quite different from yours, and if you were to get mine, or *vice versa*, there could be trouble.

My point is that bacteria have a context. In the right context, such as the human intestine, *E. coli* has a job and does it well. However, when a pathogenic mutant comes into the same setting, it can create a variety of digestive problems. When we detect *E. coli* in the environment, it indicates the presence of mammalian feces and, perhaps more importantly, it's an indicator that there may be hundreds of other fecal bacterial species present as well.

So, if that's the case, then *managing bacteria is a problem of managing context*. When bacteria interact in one way, they can be beneficial or just neutral; if they interact in a different way, they can be dangerous pathogens. Many digestive disorders have a bacterial underpinning, but the problem is typically not the bacteria so much as the conditions that the bacteria are in. And those conditions are almost always conditions that are unusual, out of balance, or the result of disturbance.

Second, for bacteria to be useful to us, context is everything. If the environment that supports bacteria is the food they eat, then managing the bacterial environment is really a food problem. I mentioned that happy bacteria can produce prodigious numbers of descendants quickly, but "happy" is the contextual part. Happy for a bacterium means having a lot of food in the appropriate environment, but happy bacteria for humans also means the bacteria are behaving themselves and not making us sick.

One important way to keep bacteria in line is to create conditions that make a LOT of different kinds of bacteria happy, but not necessarily plentiful. That is, a situation where there is a lot of food of many different types, but no one bacterium species can become super-abundant.

The microbiome bacteria in our colon are mostly vegetarians. They derive their energy from undigested plant material, which is to say, the portions of our diet that we are unable to digest quickly. Humans lack the enzymes to digest plant fiber and cellulose, but the bacteria produce enzymes that attack specific kinds of molecules making up the plant material. We can house and feed hundreds of species of bacteria if we eat a diversity of plant types which then provides a high diversity of food molecules for the bacteria.

The higher the diversity of plants in our diet, the more species of bacteria we can support and the lower the likelihood that any one species becomes super-abundant. So, for a healthy microbiome, *we must create a context* that promotes as many opportunities for bacteria as possible, and that means eating a wide variety of plant materials.

Third, food for humans should be food for bacteria. If we understand that we are not eating for ourselves alone but for the trillions of bacteria in our colon that are helping to manage our health in important ways, then it changes our relationship with food. I need carbs, fats, and proteins every day for energy and to maintain the systems in my body. But that's just for me.

I can eat my human food and think I'm eating well without providing anything useful to my microbiome. On the other hand, when I eat for the microbiome, I am not really eating for me because most plant material does not provide much (relatively speaking) of the three food sources we tend to focus on. Leafy veggies just don't provide carbs, fats, and protein in huge amounts. True, seeds can provide those molecules, but seeds may not provide much indigestible fiber for the microbiome.

So, making good food choices is important, and it should be a daily process. In older times, just eating the food we grew on the farm meant some meat and lots of garden produce. Typically, the food we grew consisted of roots in the winter, greens in the spring, and fruits and seeds in the summer. The food we ate had an annual cycle.

Today, in most affluent countries, food from any part of the year is available at any time. And that out-of-season food is coming from faraway places such as Mexico, Chile, and New Zealand. There isn't anything particularly wrong with that, but it should be part of the decision-making process. Yes, I can eat apples every day, but I should also remember that fruits and seeds are not the same as leafy greens.

And "vegetable" refers to vegetation, not to fruits and roots. Fruits are sugary, roots are starchy, and both are nutritious food sources, but that kind of food is more for you and less for your microbiome unless the food includes significant indigestible fiber.

In addition, for the past 60 years, as the world population has skyrocketed, we have been actively breeding crop plants to grow faster and faster in shorter and shorter amounts of time. And now, most of the (non-tree) produce we find in the store is grown in highly modified conditions, often in greenhouses, in non-natural, highly-fertilized environments that typically include a great many chemicals to reduce bacteria, fungi, and insect pests. Because they are grown in such a short amount of time, these foods have fewer nutrients, lower levels of fiber, and lower intensity of flavors than they used to.

The fiber and the flavors are molecules that are important to the microbiome, but many of these plant chemicals take time to be produced. Our commercially and industrially produced foods usually look quite normal, but they are of lower nutritional quality than in the past.

It is important to keep in mind that the nutritional quality *for you* might be exactly the same as always because you need mostly carbs, fats, and proteins, but the nutritional quality *for your microbiome* is suffering. And this means that we not only have to eat with a careful eye toward our microbiome, but the food that we think is good for our little friends may be dramatically lower in quality than it was in the past.

Fourth, you are not alone. Our society and potentially the human species may be in considerable trouble because of the way we have been treating our microbiomes for the past 70 years. We have been dramatically and rapidly changing the quality of our environment since the end of WWII. In 1945, we introduced antibiotics and began a social program to kill all bacteria. We did not know about the importance of the microbiome to our health. In 1947, synthetic pesticides became widely available and killed vast numbers of pest species, but a great many useful and beneficial species were also killed as collateral damage. Simultaneously, synthetic fertilizers began to replace manure and other natural fertilizing techniques and caused great damage to the health of our agricultural soils.

The number of these new chemical compounds exploded rapidly and are now ubiquitous in the human environment. Food quality is affected by the use of pesticides and fertilizers, and our personal ability to handle food is affected by our microbiome. Plastics, pharmaceuticals, and a diversity of household chemicals were introduced by the thousands from the 1950s onward and were quickly incorporated into every aspect of our lives. Through our rapidly escalating technological expertise, we are literally surrounded by an invisible chemical chaos at every moment of the day.

Today, we are all facing health problems and concerns that have never been part of the human experience before this. Our approach has always been to focus on each individual disease and find the single environmental factor that causes it because this is how humans tend to deal with problems. Find the root cause and change it. However, this time, the root cause is our lifestyle. We have changed so many variables in our environment that we cannot find the root cause of individual problems. Instead of looking for the culprit, we need to step back and consider what it is that makes humans healthy, focus on that instead, and eliminate those things that prevent us from experiencing normal robust health.

These issues are not yours alone; they are ours as a society and as a species. We have to come to grips with the fact that our medical world is lost in a foreign land and standing on thin ice (to mix a few metaphors). Our external world is damaged and that has caused damage to another world that is within us. The two are inextricably connected. However, if we accept that the foundation of our personal heath is the health of the internal ecosystem we call the microbiome, then we can focus on changing our behavior in ways that promote the health of that foundation.

Wait, what should I eat?

Most of us eat some version of the Western Diet,[7] which is comprised of highly processed foods rich in carbs and fats. In broad terms, let me redefine the Western Diet somewhat differently than you may have seen in the past: *The Western Diet is focused on feeding the human body and not on feeding the microbiome within the human body.*

As a consequence, at every turn in the grocery store and restaurant, we are sold carb-fat-protein-rich and plant-fiber-poor foods that do not support the microbiome's management of our internal physiology and biochemistry. And that means our immune

---

[7] The Western Diet is typified by high sugar and saturated fat content with low amounts of plant fiber as a direct consequence of the increasing proportion of highly processed foods. The sugar portion includes a great many calories from refined grains, especially wheat.

system and nervous system, and metabolic functions are impaired. It's not that fast food is poison *per se* and that you can't have a guilty pleasure on your cheat day, but this is not a daily diet that is good for us. It's a diet that (purposefully) appeals to our weaknesses; it preys on our cravings rather than representing a small treat or dessert.[8]

For our health, *our daily diet must be a diet that is focused on feeding our microbiome.* Our microbiome needs plants, and it needs plants that provide a lot of diversity in terms of materials. We do not need to prepare the plants for the bacteria either. Overcooked plants may be easy to chew, but that means they are already broken down chemically. We need to give our bacteria jobs, difficult jobs that require special skills, not minimum wage jobs that any common bacteria can do. To do this, we have to consider the quality of the plant foods we are eating.

For example, we need fresh (or flash-frozen) green leafy vegetables such as kale, spinach, cabbage, collards, and other greens, that are cooked as lightly as possible. We need fresh fruits, not juices. We should eat the entire fruit, skin and all, on apples, tomatoes, and grapes. The skin is important. Eat nuts and seeds, and don't be afraid of the oils. (Of course, it's important to be aware of personal sensitivities to certain foods, such as allergies.)

Lastly, we should eat plants with strong flavors, but we are breeding flavor out of our food. The food industry is now in the business of adding flavor to maintain uniformity[9] and that means the food industry prefers plants and animals to be produced in such a way that flavor is de-emphasized.

Throughout our history, we have eaten plants *because of the flavors*, not in spite of them. The flavors are indicators to the human palate of the qualities of the plant. All plant-eating animals choose

---

[8] Read *The Dorito Effect* by Mark Schatzker (2015) for an entertaining and frightening look at how the flavors of our foods are being manipulated to induce eating rather than health. A recent article in The Guardian discusses the correlation between the Western Diet and autoimmune diseases:
https://www.theguardian.com/science/2022/jan/08/global-spread-of-autoimmune-disease-blamed-on-western-diet

[9] The goal of all large food-producing corporations, especially fast-food chains, is to serve a dependable, consistent, uniform product. The MacDonald's Corporation created the business model. No matter where you go *in the world*, the Macdonald's burger and fries will taste exactly as you remember them from your hometown. This is literally a promise that MacDonald's makes to you as a customer and this is accomplished by adding specific flavors to otherwise flavorless foods.

their plants carefully and primarily by smell and taste. We do the same. Why? I suggest we do it because the plant flavors are an indicator of food quality and important to our microbiome. It is one of our ways of feeding our microbiome, and the reward for eating plants with strong flavors is our health.

Keep in mind that plant flavors are toxins for insects and other would-be predators. Many of those toxins are likely to be anti-bacterial and anti-fungal as well. If we find certain plant flavors pleasurable, there is almost certainly a good historical reason: consuming such flavors improves our health because they influence our microbiome, which influences our immune system, *which influences our survival*. It is no accident that humans have an excellent sense of taste and smell.

Our food is truly our medicine. At least, it should be. We must insist on good and strong medicine. And the best way to gauge that is by the flavor of the plants we eat. Our modern world is awash in synthetic medicines designed to solve our health problems when all the while, we are surrounded by answers to our health questions in the form of good old traditional food. The difference now is we are beginning to appreciate that we are not alone in another way – we have to feed 30 trillion bacterial partners when we eat. This was the missing piece. Knowing this, we can re-evaluate food and our eating habits and what we will find is that we have more control over our health than we imagined.

Chapter 3

We Embrace Technology

"If the human brain were so simple that we could understand it, we would be so simple that we couldn't."
                                                    -Emerson M. Pugh

How We Got Into This Mess
   The human race has always lived under the specter of impending disease and death from infections. Life today is immeasurably better than it was 120 years ago when specific viral and bacterial vaccines were just being introduced. The quality of life jumped again 75 years ago when the availability of broad-spectrum antibiotics became commonplace. Despite living in the Industrial Age, despite automation, despite slowly gaining control of our food supply, and despite our great intellect, until recently we could not conquer the greatest of our foes. The greatest is also the tiniest: bacteria.
   This single accomplishment, the development of antibiotics, has transformed the world at every level of organization, from the family to the village to the entire society. And yet, all is not well. We know a hundred times more about bacteria today than we did 30 years ago and one of the things we have learned is that we did not, in any way, shape, or form, conquer bacteria. In fact, bacteria are teaching us about how the world really works and we are now learning that it is not a one-sided relationship. To be fair, our perceptions of bacteria are based on a long history of negative experiences, but our understanding of the situation was far from complete and probably hindered by our long-standing bacterial bias.
   Prior to 1900, about 25% of all babies died before the age of two from a wide variety of infectious agents that included influenza, pneumonia, measles, typhoid, scarlet fever, diphtheria, whooping

cough, and syphilis. Another 25% of the population died of other infectious diseases (such as tuberculosis) before the age of 20, which is a period of life that is now almost immune to the lethal ravages of viral and bacterial infection. For women, there was about a one in six chance of dying as a complication of childbirth. Prior to the mid-1800s, making it to age 50 was an achievement that only about 10% of the population could claim. It should not be surprising that elderly people were uncommon, and they were special; they had survived a lifetime facing the gauntlet of hazards of the human environment. The elderly were revered and, not surprisingly, were sought out by younger people to learn their secrets to a long life.

A newspaper from my area in South Carolina, the *Horsecreek Valley News* from May 1905, reveals an interesting and probably typical view of our culture of the time. Scattered throughout the paper, surrounding the clothing ads and articles, are advertisements for a variety of rather specific products. About every other advertisement is for a life-saving or life-transforming concoction and often accompanied by a testimonial as to its efficacy. Here are a couple of examples:

Strikes Hidden Rocks
When your ship of health strikes the hidden rocks of Consumption, Pneumonia, etc., you are lost, if you don't get help from Dr. King's New Discovery for Consumption. J. W. McKinnon, of Talladega Springs, Ala., writes: 'I had been very ill with Pneumonia, under the care of two doctors, but was getting no better when I began to take Dr. King's New Discovery. The first dose gave relief, and one bottle cured me.' Sure cure for sore throat, bronchitis, coughs, and colds. Guaranteed by [local] drug stores, price 50c and $1.00. Trial bottle free.

Cheated Death
Kidney trouble often ends fatally, but by choosing the right medicine, E. H. Wolfe, of Bear Grove, Iowa, cheated death. He says: "Two years ago I had Kidney Trouble, which caused me great pain, suffering, and anxiety 'but I took Electric Bitters' which effected a complete cure. I have also found them a great benefit in general debility and nerve trouble and keep them constantly on hand, since, I find they have no equal." [local druggist], guarantees them at 50c.

The Old Time Way
Our grandmothers gave us powders and teas because they knew nothing of modern medicine and methods. In this age of progress and discovery, nicely coated, compressed tablets are fast, superseding the old time

> powders and teas. Rydale's Liver tablets are compressed chocolate coated tablets, easy to swallow, pleasant in effect, always reliable. They contain ingredients that cannot be used in powders or teas. Ingredients that have an effect upon the liver that is never attained from the so called liver powders etc. A trial will prove their merits.

It's clear from the abundance of the ads that infections and malaise were a constant concern in the lives of the local population and literally any potential cure would be given consideration, although it is highly likely that most of the concoctions were no more than the equivalent of snake oil. However, this was the tone of the times. Death was just around the corner, people of all ages in the community died every day, and any infection or cough or rash could spell the end.

In 1905, the reality of death was not age-dependent. Anyone could die at any time. Families were large, most couples expected to have many children, and this was partly a response to the fact that several of the babies, toddlers, and children very likely would not survive. For rural families, children were the workforce for food production, and many were needed as insurance for the family's well-being. In a sense, death was an understood possibility, and families fought that reality by producing more children.

Today, when someone dies at a young age, whether from flu or a car accident, the story could make the front page of the local newspaper. Such an event is noteworthy because it is rare; death at a young age is not an accepted occurrence in modern society. We have the technological tools to prevent death, even among the elderly, and we are shocked when the medical system fails. As a consequence, life expectancy has risen and risen as fewer and fewer young people are taken by disease. Now, living to 80 or 90 is a normal expectation.

From about 1900, the rapid development of water purification and plumbing systems, electrification, refrigeration, vaccines, and other technological breakthroughs caused mortality among children (and others) to plummet. With the rapid drop in mortality rates and a parallel rise in industrialization, the United States and other developed countries rapidly progressed through the Demographic Transition – death rates dropped, birth rates stayed high, and the populations grew and grew.

Moving away from the poor and sick rural areas and toward the cities and jobs was a move toward technology and health. Of course, many other factors were involved, not the least of which were two World Wars, but the transition was inevitable. And although cities are the most likely places for epidemic outbreaks, they are also the hubs of research and medicine and accessibility to technological advances that create sanitary living conditions.

The end of World War II marked a period of further technological transition: from early medicine to modern medicine, from old-style agriculture to modern agriculture, from chemical extraction of drugs from plants to chemical synthesis in the laboratory. The effect on our quality of life was rapid and widespread. We declared some diseases conquered and we declared restrictions on growth and production to be over. We declared the reach of technology to be without limit. Technology invaded our homes, and we embraced it.

Science and technology had conquered the environment, and life was better as a result. After 1945, we gained antibiotics that promised the elimination of death from bacteria. After 1947, pesticides and fertilizers promised to defeat food shortages. In the 1950s, the Green Revolution promised the end of worldwide hunger and starvation. Technology was saving us, and much more technology was on the way.

As we moved beyond the 1950s and 60s, the presence of new technology became a part of our culture and affected every conceivable aspect of our lives. Pharmaceuticals and synthetic drug breakthroughs were being introduced weekly and were revolutionizing medicine and pain management. Personal care products by the hundreds flooded the marketplace and we applied them to every part of our bodies. Plastics arrived in the mid-50s, replacing glass and metal in every possible way, and became ubiquitous within a short time. Food became "fast" and some was genetically modified. High fructose corn syrup replaced beet sugar (which had replaced cane sugar) and became ubiquitous in the processed food supply.

Indeed, our food supply rapidly became more and more processed. Grains were stripped of their nutritional value and then "enriched" after processing. Our meat supply is now a corn supply transformed into animal flesh. Our veggie production is shifting from the open farm to closed greenhouse, with the plants grown in factory-style hydroponic or "growth medium" conditions rather than in soil.

Technology has increasingly insulated us from the world to the point that we now consume antibiotics as a matter of course, 32% of babies are born by Caesarean section, and medical interventions attempt to manage our obesity. We are being promised that pharmaceutical specificity based on individual genetics will soon address every ailment we have. Technology has met and surpassed the challenges posed by the restrictions of the environment, and technology promises to never let us down.

Technology has conquered the majority of historical threats to our health and well-being and, even though we are currently faced with the rise of "modern plagues," we can be sure those days are numbered. Since the 1950s, we have witnessed an incredible rise in autism, obesity, diabetes, asthma, allergies, ADHD, lupus, rheumatoid arthritis, colitis, irritable bowels, gluten sensitivity, multiple sclerosis, Alzheimer's, and Parkinson's. Yes, these too will fall before the strength of our technology. Or will they? This is the critical question that we should be asking. What if our adoption of technology as it applies to our living environment is actually the cause of these new epidemics? What if the ever-increasing reliance on technology is responsible for the ever-decreasing quality of our environment, both external and internal? What if the disease is caused by the cure?

Is there a hidden cost to our health?

Our desire to sterilize our personal and social environments is rooted in our long and ugly history of plagues and death. The urge to isolate ourselves from nature, especially bacteria, is understandable. This is what technology has offered us in the past century, and we have readily embraced every breakthrough that reduces our exposure to a germy world, but this isolation from bacteria may come at a cost. This era of technological cleanliness removed us from the world of infections and physical distress, but may have ushered in an era of physiological distress.

In fact, the evidence for a causal connection between modern diseases and *the absence of bacteria* in our daily lives is growing daily and will soon be, if it is not already, the single most funded and most intense area of medical research in history. The bacteria that live in and on our bodies, *our microbiome*, are now being recognized as important contributors to our physiological health. And yet, those same bacteria have also been implicated, if not clearly convicted, of our previous health problems, and so we are faced with an incredible conundrum. The very thing that we have feared for centuries, the thing on which we have focused our growing technological might to destroy, might also be the thing that keeps us healthy.

We thought we had revealed the biological Rosetta Stone when the Human Genome Project deciphered all of human genetics. We then moved toward understanding proteomics (the world of proteins coded by the DNA), and recently to epigenetics (the switching on and off of genes) and other biochemical interactions between genetics and the environment, but now we've discovered the microbiome. And what a world it is!

We are finding that the bacteria in our gut may hold the keys to our health, our immune system, our normal development after birth, our susceptibility to cancer and age-related diseases, and we are just touching the tip of the iceberg. We are finding that what we know of genetics, proteomics, and epigenetics may be linked in extraordinarily complex ways to the microbiome. We are finding that interactions between our bodies and our microbiome might be involved *in both the causes and the cures* of some of our more puzzling diseases, including cancers.

Importantly, damage to the microbiome seems to be linked in indirect ways to the emergence of the "modern plagues" I just mentioned. Even more importantly – and this will be a theme throughout the rest of this book – while technology may help us understand portions of the microbiome, **technology may be of little use in correcting the damage** we have wrought on the microbiome. To heal the microbiome, and therefore to heal humans, may require a reversal of our almost total dependence on technology for solving our health problems.

In my opinion, we are about to discover how little we know about human health and how the human body really works. We are now discovering that much of what we have done as a society *in the name of public health* has been to the long-term detriment of…public health. We have waged war against pathogenic viruses and bacteria, and have saved millions of lives from premature death and disability, but in our ignorance about pathogens, we categorized all viruses and bacteria as undesirable and created technological systems for eradicating them regardless of their ecological and evolutionary role in the world of humans and other organisms.

With the introduction of penicillin and deployment of numerous antibiotics, *we declared war on the microbial ecosystem* rather than on specific components of that ecosystem without stopping to consider and understand the consequences of such an all-out assault. Understandably, in the heat of the race, for example, to defeat a childhood killer rampaging through our society, we wanted to produce a cure as soon as possible. On the other hand, once the cure had been successfully deployed, we never went back to study the consequences of that deployment on the rest of the ecosystem unless negative complications arose soon after. If the problem seemed solved, we moved on to the next problem.

While it is true that we understood that broad-spectrum antibiotics kill bacteria indiscriminately and not just at the site of the infection, we were satisfied if the pathogenic cause was eliminated. In the case of bacteria in the digestive system, we did not have an appreciation of the beneficial aspects of bacteria, but we knew that, if damaged, the gut bacteria could and would recolonize without too much help and with no real consequences to our health. Nonetheless, we knew (and suspected) nothing about the consequences of bacterial depletion in other parts of the body. Yes, we had no real reason to suspect a problem. After all, genes run our bodies, not bacteria, right?

This *genetic determinism* is the ruling paradigm of our current biomedical world in terms of both development and disease. It fits in well with our other ruling medical paradigm of *cause and effect* in the case of infectious diseases. From both viewpoints, our thinking is linear: we only think about direct and obvious connections. However, as is common in systems, indirect effects cannot be easily linked, they are often slow to emerge, and causality becomes ridiculously difficult to prove. But never mind because even if direct links between cause and effect were impossible to manage, we had technology on our side.

Even today, we remain steadfast in our resistance to the concept that the human body is part of an ecosystem. An ecosystem is an assemblage of many different species that interact with each other in ways ranging from predation and competition to mutualisms and pathogens to facilitators and decomposers. Unfortunately, our understanding of ecosystems is hampered in many ways, not the least of which is related to the quote at the top of this chapter.

An ecosystem is not just a few but potentially millions of organisms comprising thousands of species interacting in direct and indirect ways. Each species may be interacting with dozens of other species simultaneously, and interactions in one place may depend on whether (or not) other interactions are occurring in another place.

For example, the re-introduction of wolves to Yellowstone National Park created a terrific opportunity to study both direct and indirect interactions. The wolves directly reduced the numbers of deer, elk, and moose that had over-populated the park, and this was one of the main goals of the re-introduction. However, the reduction of the herbivore populations *and the damage they were causing* had indirect effects on other species in the park. One notable result was that bushes grew back along the rivers, which caused deepening and cooling of the water, which resulted in a return of trout to the rivers. The addition of wolves changed the environmental context of Yellowstone both directly and indirectly.

Chapter 4

The Importance of Diversity

Our understanding of complex natural ecosystems is not particularly good, but we have had an appreciation of the importance of species diversity for a long time. In recent years, we've begun to talk about the importance of both "vertical" and "horizontal" diversity to ecosystem stability. By vertical, I mean the importance of having the different levels of the trophic system intact.[10]

To have carnivores, there must be sufficient food, which means other animals, which means herbivores, which means plants. A lot of plants and of many kinds. A pride of three-hundred-pound African lions requires a large number of gazelles, and they, in turn, require a large year-round supply of plant material. And that's just for one of the big African carnivores. If plant life is scarce, we can't expect high diversity of large carnivores because there wouldn't be enough food to support populations of other species in the food web.

Vertical diversity is also important because it helps to prevent dominance by one or a few species at the other trophic levels. Carnivores are predators and eat herbivores and are therefore a top-down control on herbivore abundance. As with the Yellowstone wolf example, this reduces habitat damage caused by overly abundant herbivores. Without the top-down control, the herbivore population can grow to environmentally ruinous numbers, as with white-tailed deer after wolves were exterminated on the East Coast of the US. (Of

---

[10] In this case, trophic level means a feeding level. Typically, these are producers (plants), herbivores, carnivores, and top carnivores. Terrestrial systems may have 3-5 trophic levels and highly productive oceanic systems can have as many as 6-7. Humans are invariably at the top of the food chain.

course, the number of deer is reduced periodically by overeating of the food supply and by disease outbreaks.)

By horizontal diversity, I mean "redundancy" in the sense that each trophic level has many species, each doing similar things. A stable ecosystem has many species of plants and many species of herbivores eating those plants. If one species is lost, the ecological function that species provides is not lost because there are many other species filling that ecological role. We understand that such horizontal diversity (that is, ecological redundancy) is critical for creating and maintaining stability in ecosystems. In short, these are basic rules that govern the organization and the actions of the natural world.

However, even as we have come to understand a great deal more about natural ecosystems and the fundamental importance of diversity, humans hold themselves apart from the natural world. And our growing reliance on technology has enhanced that separation, but technology has in no way replaced the natural world.

Our use of technology is typically a one-size-fits-all approach. This is a problem because, as mentioned earlier, we now recognize that interactions within an ecosystem depend on the specific contexts in which they occur. With technology, we unconsciously assume that conditions are uniform for everyone affected by the technology. For example, we acknowledge that every person is genetically unique and that each of us has an ethnic history reflected in our genotype, but we tend to treat humans and the human environment as if we were all the same. We do the same for our effects on the natural world.

This one-size-fits-all approach is particularly prevalent in the medical industry where medicine prescriptions are often uniform even though drugs affect each of us differently. For one person, a 200mg dose of ibuprofen is effective, but another person might require 400mg for the same response. The rapidity at which a drug works, how long it is effective, the effective dosage, and whether it makes us sleepy or restless or constipated or causes loss of appetite all differ from one person to the next. The effectiveness of a great many drugs depends on an individual's medical history, such as childhood trauma, or current medical status, such as diabetes or recovery from recent medical procedures. Many drugs cannot be taken in conjunction with other drugs or with certain foods. Drug efficacy may depend on the patient's age or gender or obesity, or metabolism. People are highly variable as individuals, and we each have our own physiological context.

This individuality in terms of medicines is the basis of emerging technologies for managing our health based on our genetic differences. It is now a simple procedure to submit a DNA sample and receive a detailed description of many of the particular genetic variants (alleles) each of us possesses, and this can be useful for understanding what genetic disorders we might *potentially* experience in our lives. Getting a genetic screen can inform you about, for example, a tendency in your family for heart disease or cancer.

But can the presence of a particular allele tell you whether you will *get* heart disease or cancer? *No, it cannot.* It can only offer the barest of knowledge that you possess the allele and there is *an estimated probability* of contracting the disease, and that estimate is based on some number of other people who have (or had) the same allele and did or did not contract the disease. This uncertainty about how genes are expressed and how they affect us is the crux of the problem.

Let's say 100 people are carrying an allele for a particular disease. How many will get that disease? And when? And will it be lethal or disabling? There is no answer to any of those questions. The probability can only be estimated and not very accurately. Each person has a unique life history filled with a huge number of experiences that affect their health. An infinite number of combinations of experiences could potentially influence how they react to new experiences. Our internal biochemistry is an incredibly complex, dynamic, and constantly adjusting world and each person's reaction to the outside world depends on their genetics and their personal history.

The medical and genetic research world has a limited understanding of the interactions of the genes and the proteins they produce and even less understanding of how the genetic variation within humans affects those interactions. The best a medical specialist can say is "there is a 30% chance of developing this disease," which is potentially a more frightening statement than saying nothing at all. It's the same as saying, "There is a 30% chance you have a bomb in your body, but we won't know until it goes off. Until then, HAVE A GREAT DAY! ☺"

And when it comes to antibiotics, in which an attempt is being made to eradicate a particular living organism from inside a person's body, the consequences of this one-size-fits-all approach are magnified. The problem begins with the application: we ingest or inject the antibiotic into the human system and expect it to disperse throughout the entire body regardless of the site of the infection. Even when the infection is localized (like an infected finger) and can be treated locally, doctors will typically prescribe a broad-spectrum oral antibiotic "just in case."

Antibiotics are indiscriminate; they kill all bacteria of particular types regardless of the role they might be playing and regardless of whether or not they are pathogenic or are the cause of the particular medical problem. Thus, bacteria in the tissues, in the organs, *and in the gut* are all attacked simultaneously. The negative effects of the target pathogen are indeed reduced and the body's own defenses are able to regain control, but any positive effects the non-target bacteria might have been providing are also reduced.

Because we are all different, this is where the consequences become interesting. For some people, this loss of potentially beneficial bacteria can have long-term indirect effects, and we have literally no idea how that works because we tend to interpret all effects in terms of causes that we can observe *right now*. For example, if a patient takes an antibiotic series for a bowel problem and a year later develops acid reflux, it is highly unlikely a medical practitioner would make a connection between the two diseases.[11]

Same but different bacteria too?

Recent studies reveal that the species composition of the human microbiome is similar among people within a culture and becomes increasingly similar the closer two people are to each other, whether they are related or not. Similarly, members of the same family will tend to have similar bacteria in their microbiome, but only when they are living together. But these general similarities belie the amazing differences between individuals within our society.

The microbiome is strongly affected by events that occur at birth and immediately afterward. For example, the use of antibiotics on infants and toddlers has a much greater long-term effect than antibiotics taken later in life after the microbiome has been established. The damage to the microbiome early in life may not be reversible because physiological and developmental processes that occur in the infant and toddler cannot be revisited once they are completed. This research is both stunning and startling because the

---

[11] See Martin Blaser's *Missing Microbes* by for a more detailed presentation on the potential links between antibiotics and certain diseases outside of the colon.

implications are that antibiotic use in babies can cause irreversible developmental damage.

The microbiome is strongly positively affected by the food we eat, especially plants, and strongly negatively affected by the drugs we take, particularly antibiotics. These effects are influenced by age, gender, birth conditions, disease history, trauma, local environment, and genetics. The interactions of the variables that can affect the microbiome are manifold, often indirect, impossible to tease apart, and may never be fully understood. This last part is an important point of this book: *the interactions within our internal ecosystem are dependent on such a large number of variables that we may never be able to understand them*. The complexity of human physiology is now magnified by possible interactions at different times and under different conditions with bacteria that may or may not be interacting with other bacteria.

Our approach to scientific research on this unbelievable complexity called the microbiome (and this is essentially unavoidable) is that of a black box. This phrase, of course, relates to any activity in which something goes into an unknown place, and we watch to see what comes out and then try to determine what must have happened during the time we were unable to observe the process. For example, we commonly apply a medical treatment to the whole person and then examine the outward effect of the treatment on specific things such as body temperature.

Perhaps the perfect example of black-box research, and again this is essentially unavoidable, is to give a patient a drug *orally* and then examine the patient *fecally*. I say this is unavoidable because there is no way to study a human gut in real-time and in great detail or how the gut interacts with the rest of the body. At best, we can say that the drug changed certain aspects of the feces in either "positive" or "negative" ways. In fact, there is no way to study and separate direct and indirect effects in systems that have a large number of variables. At best, a correlation can be established between one action and one consequence, but it is impossible to establish causation. This is the nature of complex systems and has been captured rather well by the quote at the top of Chapter 3 from Emerson M. Pugh:

"If the human brain were so simple that we could understand it, we would be so simple that we couldn't."

From a technological point of view, in order to construct a *complete* working model of a human brain, it would have to actually be a human brain. Pugh is intimating that, to do so, we would have to understand every aspect of humanness down to the tiniest detail, but that's a level of complexity we can't possibly comprehend. We cannot fully comprehend our own complexity. We cannot know all there is to know about knowing. How much harder would it be then to completely comprehend an ecosystem made up of thousands of different species, one of which is us? And in fact, this kind of "knowing" implies linear and predictable and uniform processes, which is not the way living systems or ecosystems work.

It is, however, the way our brains work. Human logic systems do not handle probabilistic events particularly well (although the entire mathematical genre of Game Theory is one simplified approach). And so, we focus on the black-box and manipulate the inputs and scrutinize the outputs and look for hints about the nature of what it means to be human. And in the end, concerning human health and the microbiome, our efforts are comparable to Plato's cave, where an individual must attempt to divine the nature of the world by examining the shadows cast on the walls.

It is important to understand why technology, as it applies to medicine, pest control, and food production, is failing us. It isn't from an inherent flaw in the technology. Technology is inert. It's a flaw in the human application of the technology. Were we androids (i.e., robots with human form), all of our solutions would be technological, and our "lives" would be simple because there would be a technological fix for every situation. But as I will discuss next, as biological entities, our solutions cannot be technological without inviting a constant barrage of negative consequences. It's the cost of being biological, and all of our solutions to biological problems must take that reality into account.

Chapter 5

Biological Fixes For Biological Problems

*"The last word in ignorance is the man who says of an animal or plant, "What good is it?" If the...whole is good, then every part is good, **whether we understand it or not**. If the biota, in the course of aeons, has built something we like but do not understand, then who but a fool would discard seemingly useless parts?"* (Emphasis added)

Aldo Leopold (Round River, 1972)

Bill is trying to grow the greenest, lushest, most-desirable lawn imaginable and has spent a great deal of money on the recommended turf, fertilizers, soil amendments, and pesticides to ensure that grass and only grass grows in his yard. And yet, within three years, he has brown patches created by at least two different kinds of root-munching organisms as well as fungus problems. His beloved lawn looks worse now than his neighbors' (who don't even irrigate or fertilize!) In desperation, he visits agricultural advisors and lawn specialists to find a solution. Their advice? He should tear out the affected portions of his lawn, treat the soil, and then reseed the grass or lay new sod. And be vigilant for more brown patches and treat them quickly and aggressively with recommended pesticides. Meanwhile, he has to live with an imperfect lawn. These answers don't alleviate Bill's anxiety about his dream of having the perfect lawn, but he can't come up with any alternative solutions, so he prepares to rip out his diseased grass and start over.

There are rules to this game

Humans have a love affair with technology and with good reason. Throughout our history, our "problems" have been solved using our ingenuity, creativity, and engineering skills by designing solutions that are essentially outside the realm of the biological world. This one ability does indeed set us apart from the rest of the animal world because no other species can so readily synthesize a new material from existing natural materials to create new objects for the sole purpose of solving a problem.

One could argue that plants create sugar or that animals and plants generate organic polymers and these substances are novel and do not exist elsewhere. That is true, but making these substances is the result of processes based on very slowly acquired adaptations. In contrast, the human *ability* to create IS the adaptation and the substances humans make are almost spontaneous creations. They are not based on genetic recombination or mutations; our engineering skill appears to be an emergent property of our large brain mass. Our ability to physically manipulate natural substances, even to create synthetic substances from other synthetic substances, is not an adaptation but a property of our consciousness. Thus, we are different from other species, and we use technology to manipulate and remake our environment to suit our own desires.

This god-like technical ability does not change a basic rule: we must survive in a biological world. As much as some people would prefer to live in an entirely technological environment, we remain biological entities and there is no way around that. More than anything, we must grow or find food in the form of plants and animals. To do so, we have applied our skills and made uncountable numbers of tools to make that task easier. Over time, our tools for gathering food have evolved from pointed sticks to hydroponic-based greenhouses for growing plants and remote-sensing satellite technology for finding schools of fish in the ocean.

For every problem, real or perceived, clever humans have developed time or labor-saving technologies for increasing efficiency in our quest to produce food for our ever-growing population, the growth of which is a result of our food-producing prowess. We have become so proficient at applying technological solutions to these biological issues that it is the mantra of all technologically advanced human societies that "science and technology will solve this problem." We believe that there is literally no situation, biological or otherwise, that cannot be solved with a technological fix.

As I attempted to explain in *Chasing the Red Queen*, the habit of always applying technological solutions to biological problems has several inter-related drawbacks. First, technology tends to create a reliance on a single pathway to solving a particular problem which means we typically become blind to other options. If a solution works with any high degree of success, we fall in love with the solution and eschew all others in its favor. And technological solutions always seem so clever and futuristic and advanced. For many people, there doesn't appear to be an acceptable answer to the question "what other options are there?" because new and advanced is always better than old and (therefore) primitive. And, of course, the truism that science and technology will find an answer is supported by all previous successes, each one built on the others.[12]

An important part of this love affair with technological advances and fixes is that we are willing to apply them before we've really had adequate time to consider and measure potential ramifications, especially the negative side effects. The growing number of medications advertised on TV is a good example. While many possible side effects are mentioned, those are only the *known* side effects. There are almost certainly other interactions that can't be identified over the relatively short period of time that the drug was tested.

If the short-term side effects are not unreasonable, we don't think deploying the technology is unreasonable. Thus, we tend to rush to apply new technology before we fully understand its long-term effects. Without going into detail here, this is exactly the source of problems associated with genetically modified crops, hydraulic fracturing, and below-ground nuclear testing. Just because we can do it doesn't mean we should do it before we have a more complete understanding of the long-term consequences.

Second, this linear and serial problem-solving process blinds us to the fundamental principles underlying the "problems" we are attempting to resolve. Complete reliance on a single conceptual approach to solving problems prevents us from recognizing inherent flaws in the approach and from devising more appropriate solutions. It is difficult for us to *rethink* our approach. Or, if we do recognize a

---

[12] It is certainly worth noting that all successful technologies evolved from unsuccessful attempts through a long trial-and-error process, but we quickly forget how many unsuccessful attempts there were and instead focus on the single success. As an example, consider Thomas Edison's invention of the lightbulb with the tungsten filament and the approximately 1000 failed attempts that led to his eventual success.

weakness, we either apply duct tape to the fix or we attempt to modify the fix to reduce the effects of the weakness.[13]

This *technological inertia* means we will resist the adoption of a new approach mightily because we are so familiar with the current approach and have geared our entire system toward it. For example, we need to look no further than the automobile with an internal combustion engine and running on four rubber tires. As advancements in dozens of other technologies have come along, the automobile has become an extraordinary collection of radio and video entertainment, sound and climate control, WiFi-Bluetooth-GPS connectivity, and camera-sensor-automatic safety systems, but this extremely ornamented and technologically advanced vehicle remains an internal combustion engine, on four tires, governed by friction and gravity, with the sole purpose of transporting people from Point A to Point B. Even the shift to all-electric motors does not change the basic truth: the flying vehicles envisioned by *Popular Mechanics* in the 1950s remain an unfulfilled and empty promise because our focus remains firmly locked on the two-dimensional physics of the roadway. (And should flying vehicles become a reality, we will want to FULLY understand the consequences of letting everyone have a flying vehicle.)

A third drawback is that as biological systems, such as insect pests, adapt to our technology, we quickly find ourselves applying new technological fixes to the old technological fixes that are failing. This is particularly problematic when a technological fix was very successful initially and failed over time; we "know" the technology will work and we believe that we merely need to develop the next generation of the fix. What we fail to appreciate is that no matter how successful the technology was initially, the fact is, *it failed eventually*.

In essence, we are relying on technology to fix our fixes, but we aren't dealing with the underlying fundamental weakness: biological systems adapt to our technology and our technology cannot adapt to the biological systems without our assistance.

Fourth, technology is inert and is a simplistic and unstable way to work with living and responsive systems. Biological systems respond to stress by adapting, by evolving to reduce the stress, and in so doing

---

[13] Food-writer Michael Pollan, regarding solutions to problems in the food industry: "when it has a systematic problem . . . is not to go back and see what's wrong with the system, it's to come up with some high-tech fix that allows the system to survive." Quote from the movie *Food Inc.* (2008)

they become different from the "problem" to which we first applied our "solution." That is, the problem we identified and to which we applied the solution has changed such that the solution is no longer effective. In essence, we are attempting to hit a constantly and unpredictably moving target.

The technological solution cannot make appropriate adjustments to maintain effectiveness because the technological fix cannot recognize the evolution of the target. What is much worse, there is no way to anticipate the mechanism by which a biological entity (such as a bacterium) will evolve to alleviate the stress of the technological control (such as an antibiotic). There are an endless number of mutations that can cause a bacterium to become resistant or tolerant to an environmental stress no matter what the source. What we can predict without any fear of being wrong is that biological systems will adapt and technological solutions will fail.[14]

Perhaps even more troublesome than these issues are the inherent properties associated with biological complexity. Complex biological systems (e.g., ecosystems with a high degree of connectivity between a large number of species) will possess inherent characteristics that the individual does not and cannot possess. For example, complex systems possess *emergent* properties, properties that exist precisely because of the number of individuals or species present. In population biology, this concept is captured in the phrase *density dependence,* which is used to explain how and why some processes are observed only when population density is high, but disappear when the population shrinks.

For example, many of the differences between life in small towns and large cities are a function of the density of people in those places. In particular, we speak of "big city problems" because we recognize that those issues do not arise in small towns or, when they do, they are on a much smaller scale. These big-city problems include social problems such as unemployment, gang violence, long lines, and impersonal service, but also include biological problems such as epidemics, depression, impatience, and a loss of connectivity to the natural world. While both large and small human groups have these same problems, the difference is one of intensity and the rates at which events occur and the social visibility they acquire as a result.

---

[14] Grass-farmer Joel Salatin: "I'm always struck by how successful we've been at hitting the bull's eye on the wrong target." Quote from the movie *Food Inc.* (2008)

The entire subject of Environmental Science is essentially based on density dependence. As the human population has grown, so too have the problems associated with density; they become more intense and more common. And some are emergent issues that only occur when populations are large and dense. Pollution is an example in which small communities can negatively influence their immediate surroundings, but the problems would probably disappear if the inputs from the community stopped. In contrast, pollution from large metropolitan areas can affect entire regions and in permanent ways. The influence on the environment is intensified by the compounded effects of larger populations; the greater the intensity, the more likely the influence will override the capacity of the environment to absorb the problem. Thus, the pollution from a city ten times larger than a small city may have a destructive effect on the environment that is more than ten times greater.

The effect of human density on pollution from the large city has many variables and some may seem unrelated to the pollution itself. A large concentrated city population requires resources to be shipped in from greater distances than for a small population. The region surrounding the large population must support that population with food and building materials, and the ecosystem surrounding the large city will be greatly simplified for many miles in every direction. Housing developments displace the natural ecosystem and create a highly modified suburban buffer around the urban city. Air and water pollution changes ecosystem processes and reduces biological diversity as well. The ecosystem that is a human city is not only a highly simplified one, but it greatly disrupts and simplifies the adjacent natural ecosystems.

In contrast, complex biological systems can be resistant to disruption and, if they are disturbed, they can be quite resilient and return to the pre-disturbance status quickly. Complex systems are essentially buffered from the year-to-year vagaries of the environment. Most ecosystems are highly redundant in the sense that there are different roles each species can play, and there are typically many species playing each role.

This redundancy provides stability because the loss of a single species does not mean the loss of the function that species provides to the system. For example, the loss of a species of herbivore leaves a void that can be completely or partially filled by other species of herbivores. Many similar species would have to be lost before the function they provide is lost. Individual species are components of ecosystems; the ecosystem is built upon them and depends upon them, but is not defined by them.

When we apply a simple technological solution to a problem that is actually nested within a complex system, we cannot easily predict how the system will adapt to the technology. In fact, if we don't understand how the "problem" is linked to or supported by the ecosystem, then we are defining the problem in human terms without understanding its biological or ecological foundation. For example, we have used synthetic pesticides to control unwanted insect pests in agriculture since the late 1940s. Each and every pesticide that has been in common and widespread use has resulted in the evolution of resistant pest species, and this has resulted in a constant search for replacement pesticides as a countermeasure. This back and forth battle to control a biological problem with a technological solution has no ending point and is the result of an unwillingness on the human side to recognize the underlying issue.

Agriculture is one of my favorite examples. Modern agricultural techniques have pushed farming toward an inherently unstable condition: the farm is a hugely simplified ecosystem lacking diversity, redundancy, and checks and balances. The microbial communities that once supported soil health and nutrient recycling are badly damaged. The top-down controls in the form of predators that ate the unwanted insect pests are long gone, having lost their habitats and having been the accidental victims of the early pesticides. The vast acreages of single crop types have made the movement of beneficial species into the fields from surrounding habitats impossible or too slow to be useful.

The entire orientation of modern commercial agriculture is toward high efficiency and a dependence on artificial inputs such as fertilizers. The biological foundation underlying the growth of the plants has been ignored, lost, or devalued because of the nearly total reliance on technological "solutions" to the "problem" of growing vast quantities of "product." In a very real sense, the practice of modern agriculture is nearly divorced from biology; we don't *grow* food so much as we *make* it.

Chapter 6

Why The Rules Apply To Us

When we are faced with a biological problem, we rarely think about the biological underpinnings and what sort of disruption may have led to the problem. Instead, our thought process, more often than not, is to consider what sorts of technological approaches could be called upon to fix the problem. This approach tends to ignore the fact that the "problem" is likely a response to a disruption in the system, which is often the presence and activities of humans. That is, human activity creates stress within the environment, and the "problem" we recognize and wish to fix is the response of the system to that stress.

Prior to our disturbance of the environment, the problem did not exist, which implies that the undisturbed system suppressed or controlled the problem, even if it did exist. For example, the incredible number of deer-car collisions in the eastern US is a result of unusually high populations of deer, which is a result of the elimination of wolves (by humans), the natural predators of deer. So, is the growing deer population the real problem? No, the underlying problem is the lack of a biological control on the deer population in an ecosystem that has been simplified by humans. We have come up with different ways to manage deer populations, but the solutions never deal with the root problem of the lack of a natural deer predator.

The biological solution is obvious (reintroducing wolves), but not simple or acceptable, so we resort to technological solutions (e.g., hunting, contraception, sterilization, relocation, and automobiles). The result? The problem is not fixed. In fact, when the reduction in deer numbers is successful, the response by the deer will be higher reproduction rates. That is, as numbers of deer go down and population pressure on the environment is eased, female deer fertility goes up because of plentiful resources, and the result is a cyclical and never-ending problem.

Complex biological systems are more stable than simple systems and can respond to imbalances. This fundamental characteristic of a complex system has tremendous implications for you, me, humans, food, culture, and the persistence of the environment as we know it. The ability to regulate, to maintain equilibrium, is the ability to survive. It should come as no surprise then that all biological entities are actually biological systems.

To put it another way, *if survival is predicated on the ability to maintain a stable internal environment and stability is a quality of a complex system, then we should expect that all stable systems are complex*. What does that mean? It means that you and I are *systems*, complex ecosystems, even though we think of ourselves as individuals. It means that every organism is a system because survival in this world means possessing the ability to make rapid and complex adjustments to the external environment and, by doing so, to maintain an internal equilibrium.

But it reaches further than that. Throughout time, every organism has had to deal with the challenges of the environment or die. In a population facing severe stress, the majority of individuals will die and only the strong will survive. Survival means being able to tolerate the stress long enough to produce offspring who will also be tolerant of the stress. In that way, populations adapt to the stress because each new generation is composed of tolerant individuals, and the intensity of the stress on the population is thereby reduced over time.

We can view all adaptations as responses to environmental challenges, and over millions of years all species have faced (and survived) innumerable environmental challenges. The variety of adaptive mechanisms that decrease stress and increase survival is also innumerable. Until recently, we assumed the most important mechanism for adaptation was natural selection for beneficial genetic mutations, but it is now apparent that there may be more effective and more rapid modes of adaptation that do not involve the serendipitous occurrence of a random event such as a mutation.

Although we've long known about the mutualistic associations between animals and microbes (such as the cellulose-digesting microbes in the gut of the termite), we only attributed positive functions to such associations in species other than humans. We knew that the human colon harbored an incredible density and diversity of bacteria, but this was considered an unavoidable and undesirable contamination problem from living in an unclean world.

We are just beginning to appreciate how important those bacteria are to our physiological equilibrium. That is, we are beginning to understand that our physiological and even our personal happiness as individuals depends on the happiness of the bacteria in our digestive system. Their influence goes well beyond regular bowel movements and can range from developing our nervous system as toddlers to modifying our vitamin and protein balance to enhancing the strength of our immune system. Each of us is an extraordinarily complex system; we harbor communities and those communities interact with each other. Our internal communities also interact with communities in the external environment.

Thus, while we tend to think about the food we eat as being food for just the one of us, we are feeding tremendously diverse communities of species at the same time. And the community I am feeding with my food may not be quite the same as the community you are feeding. The composition of my gut community is similar to the people I live with, and it decreases in similarity as we live farther and farther apart. In addition, our genetic profiles determine to some extent what bacteria we're comfortable with and which we cannot tolerate.

Each of us reacts differently to different foods and this is due in part to the reactions of our gut communities to those foods and in part to our genetic constitution. Indeed, as we progress from toddlers through the teen years to adulthood and beyond, those communities change. The community in my 60-year-old gut is similar but not the same as that of my 20-year-old self. I've had many experiences in my life with sickness, drugs, foods, and geography that changed and shaped my microbiome composition. Where I might have had a microbiome composition that was similar to my siblings before I left my parent's house, after 40 years of separation, our gut communities are definitely different now despite our genetic relatedness.

Perhaps most importantly, the health of our internal ecosystem is dependent on the health of an external ecosystem that is increasingly influenced by human technology. As we ingest a greater proportion of processed foods, as we take more and more drugs and antibiotics, and as we consume things the human body has no prior exposure to or adaptive history with, we are relying more and more on our bacterial community to help us.

Some of these compounds are toxic to the bacteria as well and we should wonder how they are able to cope with the technological wonders we keep swallowing. How do they cope with a lack of fiber or fresh vegetables or cope with foods that are entirely digested in the small intestine with only table scraps left for the large intestine? We have to hope that the external environment is able to come to the rescue when a strong antibiotic wipes out the bacterial community in our digestive system. We depend on the external environment for providing new immigrants when the previous occupants are laid waste by medical technology. And this is only likely to be true IF the external ecosystem is healthy and diverse and capable of providing replacements. The speed and reliability of that rescue is something that has not yet been determined.

Each of us (and every other multi-cellular organism on this planet) is an ecosystem that is maintained by our external environment. As we damage and simplify the environment around us, we compromise the ability of the environment to support our internal environment, and our lives depend on that environment. If it is given the resources it needs, our internal ecosystem is capable of maintaining itself and, in the process, of assisting our ability to maintain an internal equilibrium.

The symbiotic relationship between us and our internal communities is so close and so intertwined that we lose the ability to withstand the challenges of the external environment without a healthy internal environment. What we will find through research in the near future is that we cannot maintain our internal environment without assistance from the external environment. Our internal ecosystem is nested within the larger ecosystem and there is constant flux and necessary exchange between them.

We exist in a macro-biome made up of innumerable micro-biomes, and all of those ecosystems are interacting with each other to different degrees *that we do not understand.* Because ecological principles apply to all complex living systems, we can neither pretend that we are not complex nor that we are isolated from the rest of the world.

It is also important to appreciate that our understanding is poor concerning the strength of the interactions between our body and our microbiome. Just as losing a species of frog or butterfly or large carnivore can have ramifications for the larger ecosystem, until we know more, we must be careful about the loss of any part of our personal ecosystem, no matter how insignificant it might appear to be.

And perhaps more than anything else, if we acknowledge that we are biological systems, it will be in our best interest to treat ourselves as such and be very cautious about applying technology fixes to biological problems we do not understand.

Stan has a beautiful front yard with green grass and flowering bushes. He spends a great deal of time in the yard admiring the birds and butterflies, but spends little time dealing with pests. He quit using fertilizer a couple of years ago and applies only composted leaves and grass. He waters the lawn and flower beds only as needed and lets the rainfall do the rest. His grass expanses have been shrinking as he lets the islands get larger and larger and with more perennial plantings. His problems with pests have diminished; he uses almost no pesticide and only as needed rather than the monthly commercial applications that were normal for him in the past. The numbers of ladybugs, lacewings, wasps, and praying mantises are noticeably greater. He has also noticed more birds, bees, and butterflies, but he attributes that to the greater diversity of flowering plants, many of which he planted specifically to attract insects. By mulching more and tilling the garden soil less, he sees earthworms everywhere, and fireflies have made a return to his yard as well. Stan also gets a much greater number of compliments on his gardens than does his neighbor down the street, Bill.

Part II

The Microbiome:
What Is It? Why Is It?

Chapter 7

The Little Things In Life

Judging by the frequency encountered in the popular media, it's a common belief that the human body contains ten times more bacterial cells than human cells, but is it true? Maybe yes, maybe no. The original estimate of bacterial cells in the human body came from a paper published in 1972 by Thomas Luckey, a well-respected microbiologist at the University of Missouri, who extrapolated the number from samples taken from different places in the human large intestine and from samples of feces, which seems like quite an extrapolation.

That number, ten times more bacterial cells than human cells, has been repeated and repeated until no one really questions the estimate. A more recent attempt [15] to estimate bacterial numbers arrived at a very different conclusion (perhaps). Whereas the estimated number of human cells is about 30 trillion in an adult body, the new estimate puts bacterial cells at about 40 trillion (plus or minus 10 trillion).

So, despite the considerable person-to-person variation, it would appear that the average human to bacterial cell ratio is about 50:50. However, about 25 trillion of the human cells are red blood cells which are short-lived (about 90 days) and non-nucleated (contain no DNA) cells whose main function is to deliver oxygen to the working cells in our bodies. Another 1.5 trillion cells are platelets that are also contained in the circulatory system. If we exclude the cells restricted to the circulatory system and consider only the remaining ~3.5 trillion

---

[15] Ron Sender, Shai Fuchs and Ron Milo. 2016. Revised estimates for the number of human and bacteria cells in the body." *PLoS Biol* 14.8: e1002533.

body cells, the ratio of bacterial to human cells is, yes, about 10:1 and maybe even greater.[16]

How can there be so many bacterial cells in the human body and yet we still appear to be quite human? It's because bacteria are so incredibly tiny. A typical bacterial cell is a couple of microns in size (micron= one-millionth of a meter) while a typical human cell is as large as 100 microns. If a human cell were a basketball, the bacteria would be the size of marbles. Also, the numbers of human cells vary with the size of the person, and bacterial cells can differ considerably in abundance from one person to the next and fluctuate widely from one day to the next.

Not only are bacteria very small, but they grow by splitting in two (fission) and can split every 20 minutes under ideal conditions (such as the conditions in your large intestine). In about 10 hours, it is possible for the descendants of a single bacterium to grow to over a trillion (assuming all of the descendants survive).

We might be somewhat dismayed at the rate of growth of bacteria, and certainly it is cause for concern when we are infected with a pathogenic bacterium but, on the other hand, such growth rates are the reason yeast causes bread dough to rise so quickly (although yeast are fungi, not bacteria). In our case, the rapid rate of growth means that the bacterial community can replenish itself literally overnight and can adjust to changes in our diet quickly. So, although I might have only 10 trillion bacteria in me right now, get back to me in about 10 hours when I could have 100 trillion.

So, what are all of those bacteria doing in us, on us, and to us? That, in fact, is the focus of perhaps the greatest wave of new biomedical research in history. Those bacteria are essential, dynamic, functional, protective, problematic, and tremendously diverse. There isn't one kind of bacteria but thousands, some general and some with very particular roles.

They are so diverse and so interacting that the term for the assemblage of bacteria is borrowed from the ecological literature, the "microbiome," which implies a complex ecosystem comprised of many types of species adapted to many different niches. Our understanding of the role of the microbiome in our bodies is still in its

---

[16] Some estimates are as high as 100 million, but the interesting thing about bacteria floating in the gut eating left over food is that a large bowel movement may reduce the total by half or more since our feces are about 60% bacterial biomass.

infancy, but the initial reports indicate that "important" is an incredible understatement.

We have been aware of the intestinal microbiome for a long time. Any injury to the large intestine that caused leakage into the body cavity (e.g., stabbing, gunshot, car accident) was considered immediately life-threatening because of the release of bacteria into what should be a sterile environment. The rupture of an appendix releases intestinal bacteria into the abdominal cavity and the threat of a rupture requires immediate emergency surgery.

Long before we had any knowledge of the cause of sepsis from appendicitis, the earliest microbiologists were fascinated with the tiny life forms found on and in the human body. Indeed, Antonie van Leeuwenhoek, an early developer of microscopes, published detailed descriptions and drawings of the tiny "animalcules" he discovered in his own mouth, in lake water, and many other places.[17]

Importantly, van Leeuwenhoek found a greater number and diversity of organisms between the teeth of people who did no dental hygiene compared to his own mouth, which he scrubbed daily with salt and a cloth. This diversity and variation among individuals established the presence of the microbiota in the human mouth, but also suggested that the diversity and abundance could be a function of the "climate" of the mouth (represented by van Leeuwenhoek's daily attempt at cleaning his teeth and his sample population's complete lack of dental hygiene).

He credited his efforts at personal hygiene for the whiteness and health of his teeth and lack of bad breath, but noticed that no matter the effort, he still had dental plaque and tiny organisms in his mouth. Thus, we see early evidence that the microbiome can be manipulated by our activities, but also that it is persistent.

We now understand that disruptions to the intestinal microbiome seem to lead to physiological stress in humans. Although antibacterial drugs had been in use since the early 1900s, true antibiotics were not introduced to the public until 1945.

Broad-spectrum antibiotics, such as penicillin, were successfully used to treat generic infections because they were effective against many bacterial strains, including both gram-negative and gram-positive bacteria. The resulting diarrhea and abdominal discomfort

---

[17] A nice summary of van Leeuwenhoek's research can be found in Theodor Rosebury's *Life on Man* (Viking Press, 1969). Rosebury was one of the first to discuss the importance of the microbiome to human health.

were signs that the intestinal bacteria were also susceptible to the antibiotic, and somehow this affected both the balance of bacterial types in the large intestine and the passage of waste. Narrow-spectrum antibiotics are less likely to cause these disruptions indicating a reduced effect on the intestinal bacterial community.

In more recent years, we are beginning to suspect (and demonstrate) much more elaborate connections between human health and the microbiome, including interactions with our immune system and our resistance to infection. The microbiome is not just a complex community of bacteria living on the indigestible portions of our food but a symbiotic ecosystem that is integral to our health. But how to know what aspects of health are and aren't related to the microbiome? That is, how do we separate causation from correlation? This is quite literally the multi-billion-dollar research question.

One place to start is to attempt to create a "null hypothesis" so we have something to compare our research results to. Essentially, we need a "control" population in our experiments. In the case of the microbiome, that starting point may well be *gnotobiology* (Greek for "known life"), the study of life *in the absence of* other organisms.

Gnotobiologists create "germ-free" organisms to study physical development and body processes without the confounding effects of microbes. Germ-free research has been a common way to study biological processes in rats and guinea pigs for over 100 years. In this way, researchers can observe "pure" processes without the interference of microbes and their effects. What has become much more interesting, perhaps, are the abnormal developmental changes in the test animals that appear to result from being germ-free. The largest number of physical abnormalities occurs, not surprisingly, in the digestive system with an enlargement of the cecum (the pouch-like area next to the appendix) and thinning of the colon wall.

For example, the germ-free colon does not develop the layer of bacteria-rich mucus that lines the normal colon wall, osmotic balances within the colon are altered, and the defense systems provided by white blood cells appear underdeveloped. These gnotobiology studies provide strong evidence that the normal functioning of the digestive system depends on the presence of some portion of the microbiome.

It appears that some species of bacteria assist in creating their own environment by modifying the architecture of the intestine.[18] But

---

[18] This type of response may occur in response to other organisms as well. Research on rats found that the presence of parasitic worms in newborns and their

also, it appears that there is a shifting balance between non-pathogenic and pathogenic bacteria such that their abundance and the conditions in the colon may cause fluctuations in the mutualistic relationship between the host and the bacteria.[19] In other words, *what we consider "good" and "bad" bacteria is a meaningless distinction* unless we understand the conditions that favor one kind of behavior over another.

Two ecosystems interacting

Unfortunately, because research on the human microbiome is so incredibly complex and affected by so many unknown and poorly understood variables, we will never know the full extent to which it affects humans as a species. Our microbiome is *dynamic*: it changes as we age, it changes with our health, and it changes with our diet. The human microbiome varies with geographic region and ethnicity. It is influenced by our genetic heritage. It is affected by our personal history of disease and injury, by environmental toxins, by the drugs we take, and by the food we eat.

In other words, our microbiome is *contextual*. This is tremendously important. Our microbiome is not constant within us and its functioning depends on the behavior of the host (us) and on our interactions with our external environment.

When it comes to the human microbiome, *what we know is a drop; what we don't know is an ocean.* Even as we explore the meaning of the microbiome to humans, we are also exploring the microbiomes of animals and plants, and those microbiomes are no less complex and challenging.

As researchers learn more, the implications expand and multiply. Of particular interest, of course, is how can we manipulate our microbiomes to our advantage? Can we manage human health by managing the microbiome and perhaps rely less on artificial drugs? Can we manage crops and livestock by managing their microbiomes

---

mothers stimulated the immune system and prevented developmental disorders caused by bacterial infections, and resulted in other protective changes in the digestive system. Williamson, Lauren L., et al. 2016. Got worms? Perinatal exposure to helminths prevents persistent immune sensitization and cognitive dysfunction induced by early-life infection." *Brain, Behavior and Immunity* 51:14-28.

[19] Per G. Falk, et al. 1998. Creating and maintaining the gastrointestinal ecosystem: what we know and need to know from gnotobiology. *Microbiology and Molecular Biology Reviews* 62.4:1157-1170.

and thereby rely less on chemicals such as pesticides and antibiotics? Are some of the medical problems we face today also the result of damage to our personal microbiomes in addition to the macrobiome we live in?

The number of variables that could influence the health and behavior of the human microbiome is staggering. It is difficult to manipulate more than one or two variables in an experiment and keep the experiment a manageable size; dealing with a large number of variables is often out of the question. The more variables that are included, the more likely the "conclusions" of the study will be correlative rather than decisive. That is, the researchers will be able to say that one variable is correlated with an effect, but they won't be able to say that it causes the effect, and such conclusions will be less than satisfying.

Unfortunately, the complex interactions that are typical of the microbiome reveal the limitations of biomedical research. In an effort to establish cause-and-effect and reach firm conclusions, researchers reduce the number of variables in their experiments as much as possible to test the effect of each variable on the system. Unfortunately, such a "reductionist" approach, an experiment that manipulates only one or two variables, is automatically ignoring a large number of other variables that may be equally important. In fact, a strong effect seemingly caused by one variable can be misleading because it may mask another variable that was not included in the study.

So why do research this way? On the one hand, the human mind does not handle multi-variable and non-linear problems very well. Our experimental approach reflects how we think about the world.[20] On the other hand, research on multivariate problems is slow and often discouraging and can be frustrating for consumers (or employers) who would like clear answers in a timely manner. Ultimately, this difficulty in untangling large numbers of correlated variables is why medical conditions are often referred to as "syndromes"; there are too many variables involved to say which one, or IF only one, is responsible for the problem.

---

[20] It's also a reflection of the research funding process that is focused mainly on cause-and-effect, single variable questions with grants that last only 3-4 years. And tenure and employment decisions are based on 3-5 year time increments. Thus, embarking on a 10-20 year exploratory study is a risky endeavor for most researchers.

All of this is to say that the importance and actions of the microbiome in the human body will not be clear or understood in the near future. That's frustrating, but as we'll see, it may not be completely necessary.

Chapter 8

A Brief Tour Of The Human Body

Your Skin Is Crawling
While it may make you queasy to know this, your digestive system may be just the tip of the proverbial iceberg. The microbial community in a single person's gut has been estimated at 1000-1500 species, with about 10,000 species worldwide, but the diversity of microbes so far identified in the human mouth is currently estimated at nearly 800 species[21], and diversity on the skin is difficult to estimate but may be equal to that. Bacteria do not easily conform to the concept of a "species," and because of their size, we cannot merely look at them and determine their identity.

We typically identify bacteria by what molecules ("food") they break down or by their genetic sequences. We can say one bacterium is different from another because they each decompose different molecules or we can say they are different because genetic sequencing indicates significant genetic differences between them. Either way is fine, but how different must they be to consider them different species?

Bacteria mutate and evolve so quickly that new "species" are emerging more or less constantly. In a remarkable demonstration from the Kishony Lab at Harvard Medical School,[22] bacteria were placed at both ends of a large agar tray (like a super-sized Petri dish) that

---

[21] Floyd E. Dewhirst, et al. 2010. The human oral microbiome. *Journal of Bacteriology* 192(19):5002-5017.
[22] The Harvard Gazette. http://news.harvard.edu/gazette/story/2016/09/a-cinematic-approach-to-drug-resistance/?utm_source=twitter&utm_medium=social&utm_campaign=hu-twitter-general

contained increasing amounts of an antibiotic as one moved toward the center of the tray. Over the course of 10 days, bacteria grew toward each antibacterial boundary where growth slowed until mutations to tolerate the higher antibacterial content allowed mutant bacteria to move into the next section. In only ten days, bacteria had evolved the capacity to live in agar that contained 1000 times the lethal concentration of antibiotic for the original bacteria.

This demonstration showed that huge populations of bacteria can quickly overcome incredibly toxic conditions and that mutations arise constantly, thereby increasing the chances of tolerating environmental stress. An interesting question is this: Are the bacteria at the beginning of the experiment and the bacteria at the end of the experiment still of the same species? The two strains of bacteria are adapted to very different conditions; the original cannot begin to tolerate the conditions the latter strain can tolerate, and the tolerant strain is probably not very competitive in the original environment. After a series of no less than four critically important mutations to the toxicity of the environment agar, should we consider the 1000x tolerant bacterial strain a new species?

The bacteria in our microbiome are faced with biochemical challenges in their environment every day. The digestive community must deal with every indigestible item we consume. The mouth community is exposed to mouthwash, toothpaste, alcohol, food, and spices. The skin community experiences soap, shampoo, skin lotion, antibacterial solutions, salt, and chlorinated water, to name but a few.

The spices in our foods present interesting obstacles for bacteria and fungi. Nearly all of the chemical compounds in plants that make them taste good to humans are secondary compounds that plants produce to decrease the probability of herbivory. The flavors of plants are, in fact, toxins for insects, bacteria, and fungi, and we humans consume them because they enhance the taste of our food. If the toxins are not degraded in our mouth, stomach, or small intestine, they make their way into the colon, where they may influence the environment of our microbiota. Do spicy foods create gastric upset and diarrhea? They certainly can. Is it because they do something to *you,* or is it because they disrupt the activities of the gut microbes? It's more likely to be the latter.

Fortunately, your microbiome is quite capable of adjusting and adapting to adverse conditions. It may take a day or two, but it's likely that the consumption of antibacterial substances in our food pushes the gut microbes toward tolerating those chemicals. It is almost certain that the communities in our mouths and on our skin do the same. However, it is also true that if we manage to suppress the activities of our microbiome, shift the abundances of different species, or create an opportunity for new species to invade our bodies, we are likely to experience adverse consequences.

The known diversity of microbiota on the skin depends on sampling techniques, number of people sampled, region on the body, age and health of the person, and an unknown number of other factors, including, of course, where in the world the study took place. For example, a 2009 study[23] found 19 different phyla with 205 bacterial genera in samples from 20 sites on the body categorized by oily, moist, or dry conditions. The researchers found that the bacterial complexity, diversity, and stability differed by the location on the body (with the highest diversity behind the knee). Although each volunteer in the study was more similar to themselves across the 20 locations than they were to other people, the researchers found a considerable change in the bacterial communities when follow-up samples were taken 4-6 months later.

Another 2009 study [24] sampled the bacterial community from 27 locations on the body over two time periods and reached similar conclusions. One interesting observation was that similarity between sample sites depended on the side of the body they were on (left or right). A 2013 study [25] focused on fungal diversity from 14 sites on the body and found 130 genetic types. Although bacterial diversity differed more among the human individuals, fungal diversity in this study differed more by location on the body, with feet being the most diverse. Of perhaps greater interest was the observation that diversity was *higher* on people who used anti-fungal medications and that some fungal groups were anti-correlated with other groups, which suggested a replacement process or competitive effects.

These and many other studies have illustrated just how complex, diverse, and unpredictable the skin microbiota can be. It is probably not surprising that estimates for skin diversity were higher than those for either the mouth or gut, and this is likely due to the skin's constant

---

[23] Elizabeth A. Grice, et al. 2009. Topographical and temporal diversity on the human skin microbiome. *Science* 324:1190-1192.

[24] Elizabeth A. Costello, et al. 2009. Bacterial community variation in human body habitats across space and time. *Science* 326:1694-1697.

[25] Keisha Findley, et al. 2013. Topographic diversity of fungal and bacterial communities in human skin. *Nature* 498:367-370.

interaction with the external environment from which both the mouth and gut are buffered. The skin microbiome is, to some degree, the species pool from which the other microbiomes are drawn. What remains to be understood to any useful degree is what protection, if any, our skin microbiome affords our general health or even that of our skin.

Your mouth is alive

Although the bacteria of the large intestine (colon) receive the greatest attention, a large portion of the microbiome residing in our mouth is also considered important to our health. Although van Leeuwenhoek's discoveries concerning the mouth were not accepted initially, it quickly became apparent that there is an invisible world of animals (if you don't have a microscope), and even a "clean" human is teeming with life.

The Human Oral Microbiome Database (www.homd.org) attempts to catalog all of the identified bacteria in the human mouth. The numbers are ever-changing as new samples, and new techniques reveal previously unknown types, but the latest numbers are ~800 species of bacteria in ~200 genera. Only about half of the bacteria are named, and about one-third have never been cultured under laboratory conditions which complicates efforts to identify or name them and to figure out what they are up to.

The bacteria in the mouth appear to exist as a community of sorts. A 2010 study[26] showed that although the mouth and gut harbor incredibly diverse assemblages of bacteria, there is little similarity between them. One conclusion was that the presence of specific bacteria might not be random but rather a result of interactions among species that results in a process of community "assembly."

That is, the individual species do not exist in isolation but are typically found in association with other specific bacterial species. One suspicion is that such community structure may have implications for the health of the mouth and consequently for diseases of the mouth. In other words, some mouth diseases may be contextual; an imbalance or disturbance to the normal mouth bacterial

---

[26] Elisabeth M Bik, et al. 2010. Bacterial diversity in the oral cavity of 10 healthy individuals. *The ISME Journal* 4:962-974.

community, rather than of individual species of bacteria, may result in negative interactions with the teeth and tissues of the mouth.[27]

Although the research on positive and negative interactions with mouth bacterial communities will likely be painstakingly slow, the goal will be to look for protective relationships correlated with some species and the loss of those protections when those species are absent.

As with the gut microbes, we can assume that the presence of some species represents a mutualistic association, one that provides some benefits to the human host, and those benefits are likely to take the form of protections from invasion by pathogenic species.[28]

Such mutualisms are also likely to be subtle, to vary with geographic region, culture, ethnicity, and even cuisine. Given the recent historical breakup of complex human social structures, such as the movement from rural to urban settings and the large and ongoing shifts of humans to different continents, our attempts to understand the subtleties of mutualisms involving mouth bacteria within particular regional or ethnic groups of people may turn out to be impossibly difficult.

Following our food

Our stomach is a hostile place to most living things and few organisms can survive the passage from the throat through the stomach to the small intestine.[29] In the stomach, food is mixed with acid, pepsin, and water to make a food slurry called chyme. The contents of chyme do not pass through the pyloric valve into the small intestine until they are reduced in size to smaller particles by the churning action of the stomach.

No food is digested in the stomach (in the sense that the food is not fully dissolved into component molecules), but some initial breakdown of protein does occur. The pepsinogen released by the stomach lining is activated by the release of hydrochloric acid, and the activated pepsin begins to break down proteins, which are rather stubborn molecules to digest.

---

[27] Howard F. Jenkinson and Richard J. Lamont. 2005. Oral microbial communities in sickness and in health. *Trends in Microbiology* 13:598-595.
[28] See Chapters 14-17 for more about how the BUGs might be helping the BIGs.
[29] DeAnna E. Beasley, et al. 2015. The Evolution of Stomach Acidity and Its Relevance to the Human Microbiome. *PLoS ONE*, July 2015

Bacteria and other organisms are unlikely to survive the acid stomach environment unless they are adapted to it or protected from it in some way. For example, some parasite eggs can pass through, as can certain immature and adult parasites. Bacteria that cause different forms of gastritis are able to make it safely to the small and large intestines. Bacillary (bacterial) dysentery and amoebic (protozoan) dysentery are two examples.

And there is one bacterium that takes up residence in the stomach lining: *Helicobacter pylori*. *H. pylori* can penetrate the lining of the stomach resulting in inflammation and the symptoms of that infection traditionally have been called an ulcer. However, there are no known beneficial bacteria or microbes that inhabit the stomach, and it is not considered part of the microbiome.[30]

The small intestine receives the contents of the stomach and is immediately bathed in a variety of enzymes that break down carbohydrates (amylases), fats (lipases), and proteins (proteases). The pH of the acidic chyme is quickly raised by digestive secretions, such as bile salts, in the upper small intestine, and the pH is nearly neutral through the lower small intestine. Bacteria are found in relatively low abundance in the small intestine, and the body's antibacterial lymphocytes work to keep the numbers low in this aerobic and nutrient-rich environment. If the presence of bacteria in the small intestine is a typical indicator of pathogens, the body will do well to keep that area clean.

Not until the small intestine joins the large intestine (the colon) is the intestinal microbiome found in all its glory. Once the remnants of the last meal (i.e., the parts that are not easily digested) pass through the ileocecal valve into the colon, the bacteria go to work on them. This undigested material is the only food for the microbiome of the lower digestive tract.

There are hundreds to thousands of species of bacteria in every colon. It is certainly possible that the colonization of the colon is just a natural coincidence, a sort of accidental result of living in a world of bacteria. After all, the gut environment is full of food for bacteria, the pH is neutral, it's warm and dark, and we were just going to excrete that indigestible stuff anyway.

The food material that we can't digest is durable stuff and moves through the system pretty quickly, so the chemical breakdown of the undigested food isn't likely to happen on its own. It would be natural

---

[30] Gianluca Ianiro, et al. 2015. Gastric microbiota. *Helicobacter* 20(S1):68-71.

for bacteria that are adapted to low-oxygen environments to find and take advantage of the unused resources. This is always the case in every ecosystem; unused resources do not go unused for long because they provide a niche for any organisms that can make use of them as food. However, the accumulation of a highly diverse and stable microbiome is unlikely to be accidental, and we'll consider some reasons in the following section.

Different sections of our digestive system are separated from each other and the outside world by sphincter muscles, which are circular muscles that can open and close to allow and prevent the movement of materials. The esophageal sphincter at the top of the stomach prevents a child's most recent meal and beverages from coming out of their mouth when they hang upside down on the monkey bars at the playground. The pyloric sphincter meters the release of chyme into the small intestine from the stomach.

The ileocecal sphincter separates the large and small intestines and is important for preventing the bacteria in the large intestine from entering the small intestine. And perhaps the most notorious sphincter, the anal sphincter, separates the outside world from our inside world (just as the esophageal sphincter does at the other end). Other examples of sphincter muscles are those that dilate the pupil of the eye and prevent urine from escaping the bladder into the urethra.

At any rate, our internal world is not fully separated from the outer world, and bacteria move into us and through us all the time. In fact, our digestive system is not truly internal anyway. Our mouth is the opening of a tube that winds and turns and bends back on itself and then eventually terminates at the anus. What we put into our mouth is not ever truly inside us; it is moving through us in a tube and our body extracts nutrients from it by diffusion. When nutrients are absorbed into our body from the digestive tract, it is in the form of small molecules that pass into some part of the circulatory system, but the food we eat is always technically outside our body even though inside our digestive system.

Therefore, the bacteria inhabiting our colon are not really inside us so much as being carried along inside the tube that passes through us. Many bacteria do move from the outside to the true inside, into our tissues, organs, and circulatory system. Some are escorted by carrier cells and end up in particular places for particular purposes, but others are definitely out of place and may be pathogenic. The bacteria that remain in the intestine are there for a variety of reasons, but mostly because that's where their food is.

There are several scenarios describing the interactions between two coexisting organisms, especially when one is inside the other. If one organism benefits from the interaction and the other is harmed, we call that a *parasitic* relationship. One organism gains nutrients and the other loses some vitality as a result. The parasite concept is a familiar one and many examples come to mind, such as ticks, leeches, tapeworms, and heartworms. Viruses can be cellular parasites because they make use of resources in the cells without providing any benefit to the host.

If one organism benefits but the other is not harmed, we call that a *commensal* relationship. These relationships are a popular subject for animal shows on TV. One example is the birds that use the backs of rhinos or giraffes as a perch as they look for insects that are stirred up by the movements of the larger animals. The birds benefit, but the large herbivores are indifferent to their presence.

Finally, when both organisms benefit from their interactions, this is called a *mutualistic* relationship. While we certainly don't know enough to categorize all of the bacteria in the human gut in terms of the relationship, it would appear that a large number of bacteria are probably mutualists in that they provide some benefit to their human host. In return, we provide a safe, well-stocked, amenable environment for bacteria. Whether or not these mutualisms are necessary (i.e., obligate) relationships or just opportunistic (i.e., facultative) relationships is not well known. (See more details on mutualists in Chapters 19-20.)

Just how beneficial are these bacteria to us? How important are they to us? What is the consequence of having too many or too few of them? Can a non-pathogenic bacteria become pathogenic if conditions change? Can we survive without them? Where do they come from in case we need more? These questions and more are the subject of intense research scrutiny. What little information we have gathered thus far has already resulted in several diet plans, rapidly growing pharmaceutical sales, and a growing number of interesting books.

What is known is essentially this: *a healthy gut microbiome protects us from pathogenic bacteria, provides vitamins and nutrients that we do not (or cannot) get from our food, alters our blood chemistry, stimulates our immune system, and manages our waste products prior to defecation.* Bacteria are so abundant that they make up about 60% of the weight of dry feces. That is, the mass of bacteria in our solid waste is greater than the indigestible remains of our food! While hundreds of species may be common at any one time, the majority are from 30-40 species [31] and about 30% from a single genus [32]. Keep in mind that these bacteria are necessary and beneficial and not to be confused with the disease-causing bacteria that come to mind when one is usually discussing bacteria.

---

[31] Laurent Beaugerie and Jean-Claude Petit. 2004. "Antibiotic-associated diarrhoea". *Best Practice & Research Clinical Gastroenterology*. 18(2): 337–52.
[32] Cynthia L. Sears. 2005. "A dynamic partnership: Celebrating our gut flora". *Anaerobe* 11(5): 247–51.

Chapter 9

The Microbiome: What's The Flux?

We are not born with a microbiome; we begin to acquire it from our mothers and our environment at birth and as a continuous process over the course of our lives. At birth, a baby is essentially washed with his or her mother's vaginal bacterial community, which appears to be important as an early protection from less friendly bacteria. The infant is also exposed to the mother's colonic bacteria just because of proximity to her anus. This is also important because those bacteria are going to be essential for proper digestion.

These initial sources of bacteria are in strong contrast to babies born by Caesarean delivery whose first encounter with bacteria is from the skin of the mother, which is a bacterial community unrelated to the digestion of food or the immune system.[33] Many of those bacteria are also more closely related to disease-causing bacteria.

Upon birth, our digestive system is not yet functioning, having never received solid food from the mouth, and it will slowly be activated with the introduction of breast milk. The presence of many species of useful gut bacteria in breast milk, such as streptococci, staphylococci, and lactobacilli, implies that the baby's naïve gut is transformed almost immediately as the baby begins breast-feeding. These bacteria appear to be transferred from the mother's gut to the mammary glands while the mother is in labor. This movement to the breast milk makes sense because the infant has not yet been introduced to food, and the digestive system has not been stimulated, so the

---

[33] Maria G. Dominguez-Bello, et al. 2010. "Delivery mode shapes the acquisition and structure of the initial microbiota across multiple body habitats in newborns." *Proceedings of the National Academy of Sciences* 107(26):11971-11975.

presence of lactose sugar from breast milk will require bacteria adapted to that food type.

Lactose intolerance is a common but transient problem in newborns and may be one cause of infant colic. That is, the lactobacilli that break down lactose sugar generate lactic acid in both the small intestine and the colon and, unfortunately, may produce gas that causes discomfort in babies unless other bacteria are present to consume the lactic acid. However, lactobacilli also produce hydrogen peroxide, which inhibits the growth of the common intestinal fungi, *Candida*, which in turn can be transformed from commensal to pathogenic (*candidiasis*) for people with compromised immune systems.[34] Thus, the baby is gaining bacteria that provide both an ability to consume lactose sugar from mom and protection from other bacteria that are not yet welcome in the digestive tract.

As children age and begin to eat more complex food, especially foods containing plant fiber and indigestible solids, the bacteria community grows and shifts. Breast milk bacteria become less abundant while other species become much more common. As adults, the diet will shift the abundance and diversity of the bacterial community depending on the proportions of lactose-rich dairy products or fiber-rich vegetable material or highly processed grains. How much influence the infant and juvenile diets will have on the diversity and stability of the adult bacterial community is still completely unknown.

As the digestive tract matures and is colonized by increasing numbers of the mother's microbiome, certain bacteria will interact with the lining of the colon and help to form a protective barrier. This barrier is a mucus layer with dense colonies of the protective bacterial species and it prevents other bacteria from coming in direct contact with the cells that line the colon. This prevents dangerous bacteria from penetrating the gut tissue and causing infections or invading other organs and tissues.

These protective bacteria, in turn, seem to be mediated by the presence of an antibody, provided by the mother but also produced later by the infant, called *immunoglobin A,* which helps regulate the abundance of beneficial bacteria.[35] Thus, the baby's body works with

---

[34] N.Martins, et al. 2014. "Candidiasis: predisposing factors, prevention, diagnosis and alternative treatment". *Mycopathologia.* 177 (5-6):223–240.

[35] Eric W. Rogier, et al. 2014. "Secretory antibodies in breast milk promote long-term intestinal homeostasis by regulating the gut microbiota and host gene expression." *Proceedings of the National Academy of Sciences* 111(8): 3074-3079.

beneficial bacteria to keep the majority of the microbiome isolated in the colon.

The colonization of the baby, particularly via the digestive tract, may have implications for later health. The diversity, abundance, and balance of the bacterial species of the colon are a function of our personal history as well as a function of the food we eat.[36] The ability of the bacteria to manage our indigestible food, to maintain their populations, and to avoid being dominated by invasive species may be a persistent characteristic that depends on the conditions of our childhood. For example, a diet with a large proportion of calories from sugary drinks (high digestibility) will necessarily contain lower quantities of foods with low digestibility. If the foods we eat are the foods that feed friendly bacteria in our colon, then a diet of highly digestible foods leaves very little for the bacterial community to feed on.

When we are healthiest, we are feeding ourselves well, but also feeding our mutualists and keeping them healthy. In turn, they provide services to us that influence our health in other ways. The presence of certain groups of bacteria is strongly related to the quality of food in the diet (for example, high fat/low fiber vs. low fat/high fiber). Changes in diet can change the abundance of those bacterial groups.[37]

A Beer-Fries-Chicken Diet?

What happens when we eat a highly simplified diet and for a long period of time? We have to assume that a diet of French fries, fried chicken, and light beer (or soda) is probably not sufficiently complex to support the diversity one would find in a person eating a more traditional diet that is high in unprocessed plants. French fries are carbohydrates (potato starch) and oil, fried chicken is protein and fats, light beer is alcohol and some carbohydrates, and the diet lacks fiber altogether.

In humans, simple carbs and fats are easy to digest in the small intestine, where the molecules are absorbed quickly, while digestion of proteins begins in the stomach and is completed in the small intestine. So, the absorption *of all calories from fats, simple carbs, and proteins* is in the small intestine, and little if any of that material

---

[36] G. D. Wu, et al. 2011. "Linking Long-Term Dietary Patterns with Gut Microbial Enterotypes". *Science* 334 (6052):105–8.
[37] Ibid.

arrives intact to the large intestine. On a beer-fries-chicken diet, none of the food makes it to the large intestine no matter how fast it moves through the small intestine.

The transit time of food through the small intestine is typically less than two hours.[38] Foods with materials such as bone, gristle, and cellulose fiber cannot be digested in such a short amount of time, and those materials enter the large intestine more or less intact. This is the food for the microbiome.

On the beer-fry-chicken diet, the bacterial composition of the microbiome would shift dramatically to the few species that can survive on the meager supply of food materials. As the food supply is simplified, the species composition of the microbiome would be less diverse. The restructured bacterial community would be genetically less diverse as well.

Although a beer-fry-chicken diet is an extreme example, the modern Western Diet[39] has become even less complex in the past few decades, and this has been part of the reason for the exponential growth of the fad diet market. Soluble and insoluble fibers, lycopene, resveratrol, purple fruits and vegetables, antioxidants, omega-3 fatty acids, oats and whole grains, and so on, are all purported solutions to the problem of the modern highly-processed, nutritionally-depleted diet.

We eat more processed foods than ever before, with many natural substances completely removed and many other unnatural substances added in. The complexity of the materials reaching the large intestine has been greatly reduced. Processed foods and fast foods make up a diet that is easily digested and with low amounts of slow-to-digest plant material. The typical human microbiome being fed the Western Diet is being starved and is less diverse compared to the typical microbiome of 50 years ago or that of people living in more traditional cultures.

While it's easy to increase the diversity of the gut microbiome by manipulating our diet, our concern should be for the influence that simplification has at critical periods in our lives. If a physiological process is changed, it can have important consequences for other

---

[38] Kim, Seuk Ky. 1968. Small intestine transit time in the normal small bowel study. *American Journal of Roentgenology 104*(3):522-524.

[39] The Western Diet is typified by high sugar and saturated fat content with low amounts of plant fiber as a direct consequence of the increasing proportion of highly processed foods. The sugar portion includes a great many calories from refined grains, especially wheat.

processes in the body. That is, a direct change can have indirect and unforeseen effects.

Ecologists use the phrase "cascading effects" to refer to the multiple indirect consequences that can follow an apparently simple change in an environment. For example, in humans, some people suffer from a genetic disorder called *phenylketonuria* (PKU) and are unable to process the amino acid *phenylalanine* in the food they eat. Without the necessary enzyme (phenylalanine hydroxylase) to break down phenylalanine, this amino acid builds up in their system to toxic levels and interferes with other metabolic processes. That is the direct effect.

If uncontrolled, PKU results in a variety of developmental disorders, including such seemingly unrelated problems as learning disabilities, hyperactivity, eczema, microcephaly, and unusually light-colored skin and hair. In part, this is because phenylalanine is broken down to the essential[40] amino acid tyrosine, which is necessary for the production of neurotransmitters such as dopamine, epinephrine, and norepinephrine. Instead, the buildup of phenylalanine blocks the normal movement of other necessary amino acids in the brain, and that hinders normal brain development.

Thus, *the overabundance of a single compound* in our system acts as a bottleneck and interferes with or prevents a multitude of other processes from occurring. People with PKU must modify their diets by eating foods low in phenylalanine and avoiding such things as diet soft drinks that are artificially sweetened with aspartame, which is composed of two amino acids, one of which is phenylalanine.

As our diet becomes more and more dominated by highly processed and easy-to-digest foods with large numbers of chemical additives such as sweeteners, we run the risk of starving certain mutualistic bacteria in our gut and causing long-term biochemical imbalances for ourselves. If children never have a healthy balance of foods that favor the gut microbiota, it is possible that their immune systems, their vitality, their growth and development, and other

---

[40] There are 20 amino acids that together make up all proteins. Of those 20, our bodies can produce 11 and we do not need to consume in our diet. The remaining nine amino acids are considered "essential amino acids" and must be obtained through our food. People on diets lacking one or more essential amino acids (a form of malnutrition) will experience a variety of illnesses because of the inability to produce needed proteins. This is most often seen in infants and children on low protein diets in poverty-stricken regions, but has also been seen historically in adults on highly restricted diets such as the corn-based diet of the American South.

characteristics might be impaired. It's possible they may suffer from infections more often during their life. In this sense, *the quality of their food and not just the number of calories* is a critical factor for long-term health and vitality.

The growing number of pediatric conditions requiring chronic medications appears to be related to children having compromised microbiomes from infancy. And the growing reliance on prescription medicines from childhood to adulthood may be affecting our microbiome in unknown ways. Thus, any actions we take that may alter the biochemistry of the intestine (and the rest of the body) should always be considered with the health of the microbiome in mind, and this is particularly true of the young developing bodies of our children.

Chapter 10

The Microbiome: The Give And Take

The microbiome is a dynamic ecosystem, even more so than the ecosystem surrounding us in the outside world. The microbiome (our internal environment) can change its character within hours to days versus years and decades for the external environment. The abundance and dominance of different species can shift with the food we eat, the drugs we take, or our health status. As we age, the microbiome we acquired in childhood shifts dramatically as we experience other cultures and travel, and with long-term changes to diet and our immune systems.

This exposure to more and different bacteria as we age and travel is likely to be a *good* experience for our microbiome. And it isn't just age that determines the microbiome; the geographic regions of the world have a strong influence that is related to different cuisines and ethnicities.[41] People living in more traditional styles, such as Africa, Southeast Asia, and South America, have different gut microbes and greater microbial diversity than people in the United States and other highly technological and urbanized places, and this is almost certainly related to the kinds of food each group eats.

A number of important questions remain. What determines the movement of bacteria in and out of our bodies? Do we have any control over the stability and composition of the microbiota in our gut? Are there cyclical patterns to the changes in composition? How the internal ecosystem is related to the external ecosystem, or is it just

---

[41] Tanya Yatsunenko, et al. 2012. Human gut microbiome viewed across age and geography. *Nature* 486(7402):222-227.

a matter of the quality of the inputs (food and drugs) that we feed to the microbiome?

First off, bacteria are literally everywhere. Because bacteria break down organic molecules to obtain energy and nutrients, they can exist wherever there are organic molecules. The oceans are literally bacterial soup with billions of cells per cubic centimeter; bacteria in soils are similarly diverse and abundant. Although our main concerns as humans are typically about pathogenic bacteria, only a tiny fraction of bacteria interact with humans and most of them are mutualistic or commensal. That is, they live with us or on us, but rarely in a negative way. This is just as true of the microbiome. There are perhaps 10,000 species of bacteria in the human microbiome, but only a small number are pathogenic and many of those are pathogenic *only under certain conditions*.

As wonderful as our digestive system is, it mainly breaks down the basic molecules of carbohydrates, proteins, and fats. Amylases break down starch into sugars, and we have a number of enzymes to reduce complex sugars to simple sugars, which are then absorbed into the blood from the small intestine. We initiate protein digestion in the stomach, and proteases complete the reduction of protein to amino acids in the small intestine. Fats are emulsified by bile salts from the gall bladder and reduced by lipases to fatty acids that can be absorbed into the lymph system through the small intestine. However, more complex molecules, especially those that require more time for reduction to smaller units, usually pass through the small intestine relatively unscathed.

The substances arriving in the large intestine are food for the bacteria, but what does that do for us? The role of bacteria in the colon, for the most part, is one of fermentation of sugars, which is the breaking down of complex sugars (polysaccharides) to lactic acid (lactate) to release a small amount of energy that the bacteria can then use. This activity takes place in an anaerobic environment (one that lacks oxygen) which is the biochemical reason such a small amount of the available energy can be obtained. And the bacteria are capturing that energy, not us.

For the most part, the human large intestine is not capable of absorbing nutrients, and much of what the bacteria produce is of little use to us. However, bacterial fermentation produces acetate, propionate, and butyrate, and they are involved in stimulating the human immune system.

These three short-chain fatty acids are consumed by cells lining the gut and enhance their protective functions. The proportion of acetate to propionate also seems to be related to reduced inflammation, and both chemicals interact in different ways with the function of certain vitamins, some of which are produced in the colon.

Admittedly, the production of vitamins and other useful compounds may be merely correlated with the presence of gut bacteria and may not necessarily represent a symbiotic connection. However, as the gut fauna diversity develops, bacteria begin to occupy the mucus lining of the digestive tract and this has been shown to have a protective function and is definitely mutualistic. In particular, the presence of our normal gut microbes in the mucus lining of the colon prevents the colonization of pathogenic bacteria and resultant infections.[42]

One implication of this role of bacteria is that individuals, such as malnourished children and those regularly using antibiotics, have less diverse gut communities and may have a reduced ability to resist infections.[43] In general, it appears that our intestinal microbiota may be linked to the reduction, incidence, or severity of a large number of digestive disorders.[44] Of particular importance are the new discoveries tentatively linking a compromised microbiome in infants (often through the use of antibiotics) with a number of developmental conditions and immunological abnormalities in children.[45]

Overall, it seems that the health of our internal system can be a condition of too few or too many, which is to say that it isn't just the diversity of the gut ecosystem, but the relative abundances of the different species. Greater diversity provides for a greater range of functions and provides our system with necessary nutrients. But greater abundance can be too much of a good thing by creating imbalances.

So, what physical or physiological filters act to control, reduce, or limit the diversity of the gut fauna? The first strong filter is the

---

[42] F. Sommer and F. Bäckhed. 2013. "The gut microbiota—masters of host development and physiology". Nature Reviews in Microbiology 11 (4): 227–38.

[43] Mattieu Million, Aldiouma Diallo and Didier Raoult. 2016. Gut microbiota and malnutrition. *Microbial Pathogenesis. doi:10.1016/j.micpath.2016.02.003*

[44] F. Guarner and J. Malagelada. 2003. Gut flora in health and disease. *The Lancet.* 361 (9356): 512–9. S. Shen and C.H. Wong. 2016. Bugging inflammation: role of the gut microbiota. *Clin Transl Immunology* (Review). 5 (4): e72. *doi:10.1038/cti.2016.12*

[45] Martin Blaser. 2014. *Missing Microbes.* Picador.

stomach and the acid environment found there.[46] Few microbes can survive passage through the stomach, and this greatly reduces pathogenic bacteria from reaching more sensitive structures such as the small and large intestines. This filter is incredibly important to our health and protection from the bacteria in and on our food.

The initial colonization of the lower digestive tract began at birth as the microbiome of the mother colonized the baby via mother's milk and close physical contact.[47] An infant's stomach and digestive system are immature, and the mother's contribution to the infant's microbiome is able to pass through the stomach safely. Recent research provides strong evidence that a healthy maternal microbiome supports a healthy infant microbiome.

As adults, we have accumulated a diverse microbiome through regular contact with the environment around us. Certainly, the food we eat and other forms of contact with the microbial world will have contributed new species to our personal microbiome. However, it is important to remember that the general environment of the lower gut is anaerobic; it lacks oxygen because some groups in the bacterial community consume all of the available oxygen as they break down organic molecules. Farther down the length of the colon, only bacteria that can tolerate low oxygen environments can persist and thrive there.

If this is the case, how do new species of bacteria move from the external *and aerobic* environment to the internal and *anaerobic* environment of the large intestine? How does diversity increase if one of the filters to entrance is the environment itself? This is an understudied aspect of the microbiome. If the environmental filter is sufficiently strong, then we could suspect that the microbiome we acquire in childhood is essentially the basic microbiome we possess for the rest of our lives. However, as the anaerobic bacteria are excreted from the human body in feces, transfer to new hosts can easily occur.

This is probably facilitated by characteristics of the different bacteria. Many species produce reproductive units (such as cysts) that can tolerate hostile environments, and some bacteria can tolerate both aerobic and anaerobic conditions. This allows them to move from the mouth, through the digestive system, to the colon unscathed. Because

---

[46] DeAnna E. Beasley et al. 2015. The Evolution of Stomach Acidity and Its Relevance to the Human Microbiome. *PLoS ONE*, July 2015.

[47] Ruth E. Ley, et al. 2005. "Obesity alters gut microbial ecology." *Proceedings of the National Academy of Sciences of the United States of America* 102.31:11070-11075.

of this, it is likely that children playing together represent a suitable environment for the transfer of the microbial community among individuals, and all close social groups will tend to share microbes.

We also know that the food we eat carries a wide range of microbial hitchhikers that enter our bodies even if they don't make it past the filters. Some types of food may be more suitable for transferring passengers to the digestive system, and some passengers of some food types may be more resistant to the acidic conditions of the stomach.

Dietary probiotics are marketed as a mechanism for delivering beneficial microbes to the large intestine and the presumption is, of course, that they will survive the journey through the stomach. Probiotic foods are those that possess bacteria, such as yogurts, and these bacteria (especially lactobacilli) are beneficial because of their ability to break down molecules, such as lactose sugars, that can cause digestive distress for sensitive people. However, probiotic foods generally contain aerobic species and their survival in the anaerobic colon may be limited. Thus, at this point, we know little about the food we eat and the movement of beneficial bacteria *via* that food.

There are occasions in life when the lower bowel is cleansed or nearly sterilized for one reason or another. Strong antibiotics can greatly reduce the bacterial community, as can bowel cleansing, for example, prior to a colonoscopy. Doctors and dieticians will often recommend dairy foods with live bacteria cultures for recolonizing the intestine, but this certainly comes nowhere near to re-establishing the diversity of the entire community. No matter how severe the sterilization process, it is highly unlikely that any bacterial species is ever 100% removed and the remaining individuals will quickly reestablish the population as soon as conditions return to normal. (Remember that one bacterium can produce a trillion descendants in 12 hours.).

Recent research also suggests that the "useless" and "vestigial" appendage known as the appendix may play a key role here. The appendix is a cul-de-sac that is home to a high diversity of bacteria. Of course, when inflamed, it can be dangerous due to the threat of rupture and release of bacteria into the body cavity. Physically, it is somewhat isolated from activities of the lower colon and may act as a reservoir for re-establishing the normal bacterial community.[48] Of course, the re-inoculation of the colon is dependent on the presence of those bacteria in the colon prior to the sterilizing event, and many people have had their appendix removed.

Currently, we are just beginning to appreciate the incredible complexity of the internal microbiome, its development, maintenance, health, and direct and indirect connections to other bodily functions. As with any biomedical research, the sample sizes we need to truly understand how these complex processes affect and support humans as a species are rather immense because of the diversity among the human population itself. Between variables such as geography, ethnicity, cuisine, age, experience, early-childhood exposure, disease, medicines, gender, and lifestyle (to name but a few), it is difficult to make conclusive statements about the microbiome that apply to all people.

In truth, the particular microbiome you and I possess is, in fact, unique to each of us and a reflection of our personal histories. The microbiome is dynamic, influenced by the external environment, adapting and adjusting constantly, resistant and resilient, and works in close harmony with the human system that surrounds it and sustains it. The microbiome-human tandem is an intricate partnership.

---

[48] R. Randal Bollinger, et al. 2007. Biofilms in the large bowel suggest an apparent function of the human vermiform appendix. *Journal of Theoretical Biology* 249:826-831.

Chapter 11

The Human Mutualist: This Is An Evolutionary Imperative!

Probably the most well-known and oft-repeated themes of evolutionary biology are the phrases "adapt or die" and "only the strong survive." That is, 160 years after Charles Darwin defined Natural Selection, there is a nearly universal understanding that species and populations must respond to stress by adapting, or they will likely cease to exist as a result.

However, with the emerging research in microbiomes and a greater (but definitely incomplete) understanding of the complexities of genetics, that phrase may not represent an absolute condition for all species. For any species, adaptations to changing conditions and to environmental stresses are necessary for survival in the long term. However, for two species in a symbiotic relationship where there is an intense level of interaction between the two, the need to adapt may depend on the cooperative role each organism plays in the response to environmental stress.

When two different species have formed a *mutualistic* [49] symbiosis, they have done so as a response to environmental stress. If we think of stress as a "cost" in the sense that the individuals in a population are losing energy or have lower reproduction, then an adaptation is a change that reduces those losses and increases survival and reproduction. Adaptations reduce environmental stress. In the

---

[49] A symbiotic relationship where both species benefit from the association with the other species is called a mutualism. It is mutually beneficial to both sides. A parasite-host relationship is symbiotic, but not a mutualism because only the parasite benefits from the relationship. See the box on p.116.

formation of a mutualism, we often observe one species experiencing reduced stress (a benefit) while the other species experiencing more favorable living conditions (a benefit).

The two species have adapted to each other in the sense that each develops a genetic predisposition to associate with the other and, by doing so, continues to receive the benefit of the association. Essentially, it's a situation where being together reduced the stress they were experiencing when they were not together.

When viewed from a different angle, it is highly likely that the species experiencing the original stress *did not have to adapt to the stress itself* but adapted instead to another species that helped reduce that stress. In this sense, the stressed species did "adapt or die," but not quite in the manner we have come to think about such adaptations. That is, the genome of stressed species might not contain a gene for reducing the environmental stress, but it will contain a gene for associating with the other species, and that association reduces the stress.

In the course of millions of years of experiencing uncountable environmental stressors, any response that predictably lowers the intensity of the stress will be favored. Each of these would be considered adaptations, but they could be physical, physiological, or behavioral changes.

Unfortunately, rapid evolution can be hampered by the fact that genetic mutations that may provide tolerance or resistance to stress are essentially random. There is no way to generate mutations and no way to anticipate what environmental stress may come next. Yet, a beneficial mutation has to be rather specific to the stress. This makes dependence on mutations like playing the lottery. In contrast, the ability to form alliances with other species may represent adaptive flexibility rather than reliance on chance mutations, and this may be a much more adaptive characteristic in the long run.

We should certainly expect to see both beneficial adaptations to specific stressors and beneficial associations with other species, but we could certainly predict that beneficial associations should be far more common. And over the course of thousands of generations and millions of years, the beneficial symbioses will become so integral to everyday functioning and long-term survival that life without them becomes impossible.

Consider a population of people. Each person is an individual, each has their own genetic makeup, and we now know each person has their own microbiome. Each of us walks through life thinking we are individuals when, in truth, we are vast and complicated but somewhat isolated, mobile ecosystems containing beneficial and commensal associates.

Many of these beneficial organisms have formed *obligate* relationships with us; we cannot live without each other. Obligate relationships are assumed to have developed over long periods of time and to the point that the two species have become co-dependent. Each species provides a benefit that the other species cannot provide for itself and cannot live without. In fact, part of that close dependence can mean that one species has lost a function because the other species is more efficient at providing it. For example, a bacterium could provide a needed vitamin to us, and over a long period of time, we lose the ability to provide it for ourselves. On the other hand, the bacterium may become wholly dependent on the environment of the colon and lose the ability to live anywhere else.

Others, perhaps newer mutualist species, have formed *facultative* relationships with us; we don't need them all the time, but they are beneficial under certain circumstances. An example might be a gut bacterium that is capable of digesting a certain kind of food material that we eat only occasionally.

Even *commensal* organisms that appear to benefit from being in and on us but which don't seem to confer a benefit to us may actually be beneficial, but only under certain circumstances. For example, if the presence of a non-beneficial (commensal) bacterium prevents the colonization of a pathogenic bacterium, that commensal species has provided an indirect benefit to the host. Currently, we know little (actually, almost nothing) about direct and indirect benefits and about frequent vs. occasional benefits from different members of our microbiome.

Because of the presence of thousands of other species, both mutualistic and commensal, both in and on our bodies, researchers are now describing humans as *superorganisms*. We move through the environment like individuals, we behave as individuals, and we are not dependent on the actions of any other particular individual, but we all, as Ed Yong[50] says, contain multitudes.

What we do not have to consider every moment of the day is that we, as humans, are the transportation vehicle and housing system for thousands of other species with trillions of individuals both on us and in us. The other species interact with the environment as we humans,

---

[50] Ed Yong. 2016. *I Contain Multitudes*. Ecco, HarperCollins Publishers.

their hosts and vehicles, move them through the environment and bring the environment to them. The simplicity or complexity of those interactions and the direct or indirect consequences to our health are almost completely unknown.

This is a difficult and exciting conundrum to consider and explore. As humans, we think we are interacting with the external environment, but are we interacting with the environment as individuals or as ecosystems? Is it our microbiome that is interacting and we are just the beneficiaries of that interaction? A delightful and squishy example of what I mean is the cow. Everyone knows cows eat grass (or are supposed to), but do they really *eat* grass in the same sense that we eat our food? Actually, no, they don't.

The cow *consumes* grass by chewing and swallowing, but the grass goes into that 25-gallon fermentation vat called the rumen, the first of the four stomach chambers. In the rumen, trillions of bacteria digest the nutrients contained in the grass and provide energy molecules for the cow (called short-chain fatty acids or SCFA). In other words, the cow feeds its bacteria with grass and the bacteria feed the cow with SCFA. Thus, the daily chore of a cow is to move through the large external macrobiome collecting and fragmenting grass to keep its microbiome healthy and happy, which in turn keeps the cow healthy and happy.

We also interact with our environment, and some aspects of our microbiome are interacting directly and more intimately with the world around us than we are. Undoubtedly, our primary interaction with the external environment is through the food we eat and the liquids we drink as we move materials from the external ecosystem to the internal ecosystem. However, when we are eating a "healthy" diet, to what extent are we feeding the internal ecosystem, which in turn feeds us and protects us? How important is it to eat certain foods and thereby feed certain species of bacteria?

The majority of our direct interactions with the environment largely involve protecting our insides from the outside. However, the microbiome does not necessarily distinguish direct and indirect and inside and outside according to the same criteria. So, a more important question may be to ask *how important is that flow of information* (mostly food, but also other bacteria) from the ecosystem of the outside world to the ecosystem of the inside world?

Our movement through the environment results in direct encounters for some microbiome species because of changes in the heat, moisture, and chemicals on the skin of the human transport system. Our skin is both our first line of defense and home to a vast array of microscopic organisms populating our outer surfaces. They experience what our skin experiences, yet the skin is their home habitat rather than merely a protective layer. The species populating our skin are able to tolerate the conditions that humans are able to tolerate because they are adapted to that range of conditions. Nonetheless, humans experiencing different habitats and climates around the world are likely to possess a regional subset of the much larger possible microbial community. For example, a person living on the coast will have a different skin microbiome than a person living around farmlands or in the mountains.

How geographic variation interacts with human genetics, particularly ethnicity, has been described in a small number of studies, but we have little to no understanding of the possible implications. It may turn out that the skin microbiome does little else than prevent unwanted species from landing and establishing. If certain species are well adapted to life on our skin, new arrivals will have a hard time displacing the residents. If a new arrival is a potential pathogen but is displaced by the local fauna, this is an unquestionable beneficial consequence of a healthy skin microbiome. In contrast, some forms of dermatitis may reflect an inability to protect our skin from invasive and dangerous new species of microbes.

In contrast to the skin microbiome, the bacteria community in the large intestine will experience the external environment through the food we eat as well as the antibiotics, pharmaceuticals, preservatives, and other chemicals we consume. A person with a uniform and unwavering diet, particularly one low in plant materials, will have a less diverse community than a person with a varied diet that includes a diversity of plants. Many of the bacteria that favor particular food items are predicted to be carried into the digestive tract by that food.[51]

Certain foods will favor specific bacteria while other bacteria are generalists and can live on a variety of food items. For example, foods with lactose sugar are rather specific and favor the growth of *Lactobacillus* species in our digestive system, whereas high-fiber foods are rather common and favor *Bacteroides* species capable of fermentation and the breakdown of complex plant molecules.

---

[51] This avenue of research is just getting underway and will be a painfully slow process. To learn MUCH more, the Human Food Project/American Gut is a good starting point: http://humanfoodproject.com/americangut/

When a diet changes dramatically from one food type to another, say from high-carbohydrate foods to high-fiber plant foods, the composition of the bacterial community will shift rapidly. Those species that favor the new foods will grow in abundance, and those that are less competitive for that food type will decrease. These shifts increase digestive efficiency and the changes to the composition of the community can take less than 24 hours.

Of course, these responses to changes in diet are complicated by the drugs we take and other chemicals we consume. We know that antibiotics are more or less specific to bacteria and may greatly diminish our microbiome populations. Much less is known about how other non-antibiotic yet powerful drugs intended for managing, for example, depression, blood pressure, or inflammation, may affect all or part of the microbial community.

There are many aspects of food quality that can influence bacterial-assisted digestion, and some may be subtle. We provide food sources for our microbiome with every meal, but we may also introduce new genetic strains or species of *Lactobacillus* that may compete with the ones already in our system. The newcomers may be better for us by being more efficient at converting lactose sugar. If they are better competitors, we would expect them to take over.

Research on obesity is now indicating that the microbiome of obese people differs from that of non-obese people. In particular, the "obese microbiome" appears to be more efficient at extracting calories from food. That is, obese people may be getting more calories from the same food as non-obese people. This research clearly suggests that the different strains or species of bacteria being favored in different people is contextual, and this has consequences for human health. In this case, it suggests that the "obese microbiome" is more competitive because it's more efficient at obtaining "food."

The bacterial community is responsive and dynamic, and that is an important trait of diverse communities because of the constant interactions with the environment that lead to the need for adjustments of one kind or another. If we experience or even encourage shifts in food quality, we need a shift in bacterial composition to accommodate the digestive requirements of those new foods.

Historically, the regular shift in food quality from one season to another was a definitive aspect of human life, especially for hunters and gatherers but also for farming communities. The possession of a microbiome capable of accommodating such dietary variation, particularly for an omnivorous diet, may be *the single most important adaptation* for the human species. Such a microbiome, by necessity, must be complex and capable of rapid shifts in the abundance of bacterial species.

Herbivores also, by necessity, must have complex digestive systems to deal with the slow-to-digest foodstuff they eat. However, because herbivores like deer eat a predictable diet of their favorite plants, we would expect their bacterial communities to be relatively stable and consistent over time. In contrast, animals adapted for a carnivorous diet have simpler microbiomes because of the relative ease with which meat and other animal proteins can be digested and the lack of plant materials.

The omnivorous human must possess digestive flexibility, and this is accomplished not with adaptations for a diversity of digestive enzymes, but with adaptations to possess a diversity of digestive assistance from bacteria. By possessing such digestive flexibility and by carrying our highly diverse digestive community with us, our ability to move from place to place through the seasons and over the years must have been greatly facilitated. Thus, we have to think that the possession and maintenance of a highly diverse microbiome is an essential adaptation for the omnivorous human.

Chapter 12

The Human Mutualist: Guidelines For Symbionts

The origin of mutualistic systems, such as our microbiome, is lost to the distant past, but it almost certainly did not begin as a friendly encounter. Let's define a mutualism as a *symbiotic relationship between two organisms that provides a benefit for both species and leads to increased survival and successful reproduction* (fitness). Like all adaptations, the formation of a mutualism is an adaptation to alleviate an environmental stress. Such an outcome would only occur in a situation where environmental stress was lowering survival and fitness for the individuals in a population, and the formation of a mutualism provided relief from that stress.

To be clear, the process of *adapting is not a desirable or welcome process* because it involves high mortality in the population over a relatively short period of time. That is, if a population is adapting to its environment, that means an intense stress is killing a large portion of the population, and only the strong are surviving long enough to reproduce. Those survivors must pass on traits that help them survive the stress to their offspring, and that results in a larger proportion of the next generation being more capable of tolerating the stress. In this way, the population recovers from the stress by producing new generations of stronger and more tolerant individuals.

In other words, *a population that has successfully adapted to an intense environmental stress has just experienced a traumatic episode* that involved significant mortality of relatively young victims. No population *wants* to adapt because the process of adaptation requires high mortality, and only the strong survive. On the other hand, adaptation is a positive outcome because it means the individuals in the subsequent generations are better able to survive the difficult conditions experienced in that environment.

Environmental stress, whether through competition for resources or protection from predators, leads to adaptive responses in the stressed organisms, but which is easier – a mutation for tolerance of the stress or forming a mutualism?

If we consider an adaptation to avoid predation, it could be that a series of fortunate mutations leading to a positive physical change (such as a new form of defense) is more difficult or time-consuming than a favorable association with another organism already possessing a useful defense. The severity of the stress may be a critical component in favoring mutualisms over gene-based shifts in body morphology.

If the time available for "adapting or dying" is short, the mutations for survival *must already exist* in the population, and the probability of this is based on the population being large and genetically diverse. In contrast, the creation of a mutualism with another species may be facilitated by having two genomes to draw on and by previous ecological interactions between the two species. A mutualism is favored by simply shifting the cost of a previous association from negative or neutral to positive.

Larger organisms, such as humans, are faced with the need to adapt to shifting climates or colonizing unfamiliar habitats such as high elevation or high latitude regions with unfamiliar types of food or novel diseases. As an example of the possible pathway that leads to bacterial symbiosis and possibly a mutualism with human biology, let's consider infection by a lethal pathogen.

After infection by a pathogen, our body experiences the rapid growth of the pathogenic species, perhaps a bacterium, and we are unable to control that growth; it overwhelms our defense systems and we get sick. When we, a naïve population, encounter a new pathogen, the bacterium is likely to be highly virulent, meaning it experiences very rapid growth once it has infected us because we have no specific mechanism for slowing that growth. It's a dangerous situation because we have no history with the bacterium and, therefore, no way to defend against it. We get sick, we cannot prevent it from spreading through the population, and we have an epidemic on our hands. The bacteria grow rapidly and in huge numbers within each infected individual, and as the disease spreads through the population, large numbers of people die prematurely.

Epidemics spread for three main reasons. First, a large and dense population will have a large number of people susceptible to a new disease or a new strain of an old disease. The new bacteria spread easily in large populations because so many people come into contact with each other, and few of them have any defenses against the infection. The pathogen can easily jump from one defenseless individual to another. Disease outbreaks are far more likely to occur in cities where aggregations of people occur for many different reasons and where transportation hubs bring people together from around the region and the country. Thus, a new disease is more likely to appear in places where it is easy to spread, that is, in dense populations with lots of susceptible people.

Second, if transmission is quick or uncomplicated, the bacteria will spread from one person to another readily. For example, if a handshake or a kiss on the cheek is sufficient, then the disease spreads quickly. If contact with saliva or sputum is necessary and a sick person must cough on another person, the rate of spread is slower because that contact is less likely. If blood or lymph contact or exchange is a requirement, then the pathogen will spread even more slowly because such contact only occurs under rather specific conditions. Thus, the manner and likelihood of transmission are critical. For this reason, medical researchers are often more concerned about diseases that are easy to spread, even if the difficult-to-spread diseases are far more lethal.

Third, the period of time that an infected person is infectious to other people determines the window of opportunity for the bacteria to move from one person to another. For example, in the case of the flu, my family doctor may advise me to remain at home for 24 hours after the symptoms disappear. At that point, there is a low likelihood of being infectious. Those flu-sufferers who insist on going to work or to public places while they are infectious will continue to spread the disease when they make contact with susceptible individuals. And obviously, diseases that are infectious before the symptoms appear or after the symptoms have disappeared are the most dangerous.

Thus, diseases spread most rapidly, and epidemics occur most commonly when there is frequent contact between people, transmission is uncomplicated, and infectious periods are long or the infection is hard to detect.

When a disease is spreading rapidly, the bacterium has no difficulty moving from one host to another. Transmission is rapid among the many susceptible hosts, and this favors the strains of the bacteria that are capable of reproducing and growing the fastest, which is to say the most virulent strains are favored. Conditions that favor virulence are favoring the dangerous strains of the bacteria, which will come to dominate the bacterial population because the conditions favor their spread the most.

Think of it as a race in which the strain that reproduces the fastest is the winner. If the number of susceptible individuals is large, if the contact rate between individuals is high, or if the rate of transmission of the bacterium between individuals is high, then those bacteria that spread easily and grow rapidly in number will dominate the population.

From the bacterial point of view, it really doesn't matter if the sick individual dies as a result of the infection as long as the disease has been transmitted to the next person before the victim dies. This is a key element in epidemic situations; when conditions support an epidemic, the conditions are favoring the most dangerous strains of the pathogen.

However, all epidemics peak and subside. As the epidemic progresses, the number of susceptible individuals goes down because more and more of the population have already had the disease (and survived or died) and the spread of the bacterium from one host to another becomes a much slower and less frequent process. That is, the encounter rate with susceptible individuals goes down, and the prospect of transmission of the disease goes down; therefore, the likelihood of an infectious individual coming in contact with a susceptible individual goes down.

A key element of this process is that the bacteria must remain in each host for a longer period of time before being transmitted to a new host. As these conditions develop, which they do in every serious epidemic, those fast-growing strains of bacteria that were favored initially and that kill the host quickly now face a critical obstacle: they might kill their host before they are able to jump to a new host and when the current host dies, the highly virulent strains of bacteria die too. As an epidemic matures, the strains of bacteria that are favored are those that grow somewhat slower, kill their host more slowly, and are able to stay in their host longer before being transmitted to a new host.

There are two variables interacting as this goes on. First, the bacterial strains that come to dominate the population are those that are slower growing and less lethal. That is, the dominant strains are not causing the disease to occur as rapidly in the host. A second variable is that the host's immune and defense systems are not as easily overwhelmed by the weaker infection and are able to mount a counterattack or at least hold off the assault. Essentially, the slower-growing bacterial strains experience an environment that fights back.

Under these conditions, the infection becomes a sort of cat-and-mouse game where the bacteria must persist long enough to be transmitted to a new host while the current host's defense systems are attempting to control the bacteria before they kill the host.

In short, the longer it takes for the bacteria to be transmitted, the more benign the infection becomes because it cannot afford to kill the host before transmission happens. If it does, that strain of the bacteria eliminates itself from the population, and only the weaker strains that do not kill their host as quickly can survive. If we understand the evolutionary tug-of-war between host and pathogens, it is easy to see why new diseases with which we have no experience are so dangerous,[52] but diseases that have been around for many years, even centuries, tend to be relatively benign or only problematic for people with weakened immune systems.

While this change does not necessarily result in a mutualism between the host and the pathogen, it is useful to remember that the less-virulent pathogen remains in a battle with the host. The pathogen remains in the host population, exacting an energetic cost by forcing a defensive response, and the host cannot completely eliminate the pathogen, which is adapting to the host defenses. Nonetheless, the eventual détente creates a situation wherein the host and the pathogen are in an uneasy relationship. If the external conditions change such that the number of susceptible hosts in the population increases and the contact rate between hosts increases, the conditions are right for more virulent strains of the pathogen to proliferate and start a new epidemic. Indeed, the conditions are right for virulent stains of other pathogens to proliferate as well.

This resident-pathogen situation creates conditions that could favor a mutualistic relationship between the host and the pathogen if the conditions were to change. Low-level infections take an energetic toll on the host because of the need to constantly fight off the pathogen and because the pathogen takes energy from us. If the environmental conditions were to change, the balance of power would also change: we could lose the fight and get sick, or we could vanquish the enemy.

---

[52] For example, a novel coronavirus such as SARS-CoV-2.

However, if the environment were to change such that a new dangerous pathogen was introduced, the cost of having the resident pathogen could become a benefit if its presence protected its host from infection from the newly arriving, more lethal pathogen. If a pathogen is highly competitive against other pathogens and by doing so protects the host to some degree from new infections, the result is, by definition, a mutualism. It is also possible that the defense mechanisms for controlling the resident pathogen may make the host less susceptible to other pathogens. In this case, the presence of the resident pathogen makes the host's defenses stronger by being constantly activated.

In such a scenario, the presence of the pathogen could become a benefit. The pathogen benefits by protecting the host from other pathogens, and the host benefits by having higher survival, lower costs, and higher eventual fitness. Such a mutualism does not require novel mutations and genetic adaptation on the part of the host but just a shift in the net value of a previously existing association. (The reasons why this will work best in large organisms, such as humans, are discussed in the chapters on Bigs and Bugs.)

What Is A Mutualism?

A mutualism is defined as any interaction between two species where both sides benefit from the interaction. Mutualisms are not necessarily constant, and many depend on the conditions experienced by each side of the equation. "Obligate" mutualisms are so close and integral to survival that the two species cannot be separated, and each species depends on the relationship. For example, *Symbiodinium* algae live in the tissues and provide nutrients to tropical corals while receiving physical protection from the coral.

Such tight associations are probably very old, and the two species have evolved to the point that critical functions have been assumed by one of the species and have been lost by the other species. The Theory of Endosymbiosis suggests that the mitochondria in all animals and plants and the chloroplasts in plants are examples of ancient mutualisms formed by single-celled organisms and that these mutualisms are now fundamental to the biochemical processes of both organisms.

On the other hand, there are "facultative" mutualisms in which the association between the species is not a requirement for survival, but the interaction provides a benefit that increases the probability of survival *under certain conditions*. Under the right conditions, the individuals participating in the mutualism are more likely to survive or prosper than those that do not.

Facultative mutualisms are interesting from ecological and evolutionary perspectives because they tend to vary in space and time. There will be times when the mutualism is a good idea and times when it is not, and there will be places where it is a good idea and places where it is not. That is, under certain environmental conditions, the benefit of the association will outweigh the cost, but that ratio may change as the environmental conditions change.

For example, certain spiders form social aggregations when food is abundant. This has been explained this way: when food is abundant, the cost of spinning an individual web to catch one's own food is outweighed by the benefits obtained from a much larger collectively-spun web but having to share the food. However, when the food resources become scarce, fewer prey are captured in the communal web, and the cost-benefit ratio shifts back to favoring the individual web and not sharing the food. The spiders disperse, become solitary, and do not share their webs or their prey.

Some plants, particularly legumes, will form nodules on their roots in low nutrient soils. Colonies of bacteria in the nodules provide nitrogen compounds to the plant and the plant provides carbon to the bacteria. However, in fertile soils, the plants will resist colonization of the roots by the bacteria because nitrogen is readily available in the soil. Having the bacteria in the roots is beneficial when nitrogen is needed but becomes an unnecessary burden (i.e., the plant still loses energy to the bacteria) when nitrogen is available at no cost to the plant.

Mutualistic interactions are the subject of a great deal of fascinating research. Essentially, facultative mutualisms are based on cost-benefit analyses in the sense that organisms must evaluate the benefit received against the cost that must be borne. Organisms with adaptations for making the best choices as conditions change from being more costly to more beneficial, and *vice versa*, are more likely to thrive and produce more offspring.

Natural selection helps organisms make adaptive economic choices in a world of limited resources. When conditions remain stable for long periods of time and the costs are predictable, obligate mutualisms are favored because the benefits derived from the mutualism are stable. Understanding the give and take of mutualistic relationships has interesting applications in many areas of human and non-human research, such as sociality, philanthropy, shared risk, predation avoidance, mating choices, herd size, genetic relatedness, and food sharing.

Chapter 13

The Human Mutualist: From Costs To Benefits

The Human Mutualist: From costs to benefits

From the previous example of how symbioses with bacteria might form, consider the huge number of bacteria in our internal ecosystem that do not cause death or even ill-health. Did they evolve from pathogenic forms into benign forms that developed a symbiotic or even mutualistic interaction with our bodies?

Let's suppose a previously dangerous bacterium evolved another function that was useful to us. If a pathogen evolved mechanisms for defending itself from the host's defenses and was able to extract sufficient resources from the host to survive, then it essentially created a niche for itself in the host's ecosystem. Once in such a niche, the bacterium would also have to defend itself from the proliferation of other pathogens that could displace it from its niche. By doing so, it would essentially be protecting the host from those pathogens too. If the presence of one pathogen prevented the invasion by other more dangerous pathogens, the first pathogen, by default, can be viewed as a mutualist under conditions where new infections are likely. (Nevertheless, when other external threats are not present, the resident pathogen could still exact a cost higher than the value of the benefit.)

From an evolutionary perspective, this is intriguing. Such an arrangement means that if a sub-lethal pathogen evolves a function that provides a defensive benefit to the host, *the host essentially gains a new function*. The new function will be derived from the pathogen's genome, not the host's genome. If the new function is sufficiently beneficial, it will offset the negative cost of the pathogen, that is, of having the pathogen present within the host. In such a case, the mutualism will be favored and will persist. The benefit to the host will depend on *controlling but not eliminating* the pathogen. The virulence of the pathogen will remain low and will probably decline over time.

If a new defensive function provided by a microbe, such as a pathogen, is superior to an existing defensive function of the host, the host's innate defensive function is redundant and may become obsolete. How could the pathogen provide a superior defensive function? It depends largely on the difference between the growth rates of human cells and bacterial cells. We know that bacteria can produce prodigious numbers of new cells in a short amount of time and every new bacterium is a complete individual. On the other hand, human cells divide much more slowly and have limited functionality because cells in the human body represent particular tissue types.

If certain biochemical (immune) defenses of humans are dependent on cell proliferation, it is possible that bacteria can provide a faster defensive response. We know that highly virulent bacteria can overwhelm human immune defenses and this is based on bacterial cell growth rates. Thus, the rapid response of a mutualistic bacterium to an environmental threat could outwardly appear to be a flexible defensive response of the host.

If the survival and health of the host is a highly beneficial condition to the bacterium, then protecting the health of the host becomes an evolutionary benefit, and this will be expressed as a mutualistic interaction. (See the section on "Of Bigs and Bugs")

The huge numbers of bacteria in the human microbiome did not all start as pathogens that evolved into mutualists protecting the host environment. However, it is certainly possible that initial bacterial mutualisms created an environment that was conducive to further colonization by other bacteria. That is, if the environment of the early digestive system was generally hostile to certain bacterial types, the evolution of an initial mutualism would have created a less-hostile environment in general.

An example would be the reduction of oxygen levels in the large intestine by early aerobic colonists that facilitated the survival of anaerobic bacteria as later colonists. This change in conditions has been noted in the initial colonization of newborn babies as the lactobacilli are carried by mother's milk to the large intestine. Because the baby's digestive system has not been activated and is incapable of breaking down lactose, the process of digesting lactose sugar is dependent on bacteria.

Lactobacilli are tolerant of low oxygen levels, but the environment in the colon becomes more anaerobic soon after bacteria take up residence and begin breaking down large food molecules, which is an oxygen-consuming process. Such a modification of the internal environment could then facilitate further colonization, creating conditions favoring mutualisms with anaerobic bacteria, and thereby encouraging the eventual development of a complex internal ecosystem.

It is not necessary that all members of the ecosystem contribute equally to the health of the host, and many species are likely to take advantage of the food resources in the digestive system of the host. This can be either a parasitic situation if it deprives the host of needed resources or a commensal situation if the host is unaffected by the presence of the non-mutualist. Both scenarios are likely.

Hitchhikers are unavoidable in any large and complex system, but if the parasitic species are low in abundance and do not trigger a defensive response from the host *or from the other members of the microbiome*, then they can become part of the normal functioning of the ecosystem. However, this is likely to be the case only when non-beneficial species remain in relatively low abundance. From an ecological perspective, this is how bacteria such as *Clostridium difficile* and *Staphylococcus aureus* can be normal residents in the colon.

Regardless of the beneficial, commensal, or parasitic nature of the microbial inhabitants, all species gain by protecting the integrity of the system. That is, if the internal environment is threatened, then the inhabitants are threatened.[53] We should not be surprised, then, that for internal ecosystems, such as the microbiome, where the survival of the resident species is dependent on the health of the system, those species will provide defensive functions that support the integrity of the system. These defensive functions should not only favor the host but should have a regulatory effect on the other species in the community.

In that sense, the healthy ecosystem is self-regulating through negative feedback that limits the growth or dominance of any one species. It's worth noting that regulation of dominance can also be accomplished merely by a change in the resource base. That is,

---

[53] Obviously, this is not true for pathogenic species. The integrity of the ecosystem is only relevant insofar as the transmission of the pathogen to the next host is facilitated.

frequent changes in the quantity and quality of the food eaten by the host, particularly foods that favor greater microbial diversity, will prevent dominance by one or a few species. Why is this important?

In complex ecosystems, dominance by one species is rare and typically indicates an imbalance in the structure of the system. For example, dominance implies that one species is capable of being competitively superior across the range of available resources, but that would mean being able to outcompete all other species, including the specialist species. In a system with a diversity of both resources and species, this should not occur.

When the resource base is simplified, or the species composition of the ecosystem has been simplified, the conditions are favorable for one or a few species to dominate and even eliminate less competitive species or those lacking sufficient resources. High species diversity typically reflects high resource diversity and should also favor both generalist and specialist species, and the presence of both types will prevent any one of them from dominating the system.

One implication of this is that *species diversity is probably a vital characteristic for the maintenance and stability of an internal ecosystem.* In a microbiome, there is a need for the resident species to recolonize after depletion, to exchange with and stay up to date with the external ecosystems, to respond to changing conditions, to compete with other species, to specialize for resources, and to take quick advantage of new resources. All of these response functions favor species diversity and redundancy, and resource specialization.

In short, *a healthy and stable microbiome is a diverse microbiome that is being supported by a diverse resource base,* and such a microbiome will be efficient at digesting food and supportive of the host system. In addition, species diversity and redundancy means that the loss of one or more species will not greatly disrupt the system because other species are available to fill the roles of the lost species. *This then leads to greater resilience because the system can rebound quickly from a serious disruption.* Again, for human systems that are inherently limited in their response flexibility, the presence of a mutualistic and diverse microbial community will provide necessary functions for maintaining a healthy and responsive system.

In summary, the availability of the microbial genomes for providing new abilities to the host means that *humans are more complete ecosystems when we have a healthy microbiome* to support us.

Chapter 14

Of BIGs And BUGs: Why Size Does Matter

For professors who teach evolutionary biology, the question will always arise: Have humans adapted to the environment? Answer: Yes, of course, they have. Humans, like any species, have a long unbroken history of successfully adapting to the stresses and challenges of the environment. We show those adaptations in a number of physical attributes, especially in our biochemistry and immune systems. But are humans adapting to the current environment? The short answer is, no, not really.

The question usually comes up during conversations about epidemics such as HIV/AIDS and whether humans will become resistant or immune to the HIV infections. The answer is not really one of whether we are capable of evolving resistance (yes, we are), but whether it will actually happen, and that answer is no, it won't. What is far more likely is that HIV will adapt to us for the reasons explained in the previous chapter.

The explanation of why we won't adapt requires going over some basics of evolutionary biology. Essentially, the problem is this: *we just don't have the time to adapt* to HIV, a coronavirus, or any other pathogen in our environment. The rate of evolution is the time necessary for a population to adapt to a particular stress in the environment. That time depends on several variables.

First, we have to possess, somewhere in the population, the genetic variation needed to tolerate a stress that is highly lethal. That variation will be a mutation that a number of people unknowingly carry with them, buried in their chromosomes, waiting for the opportunity to be expressed. As an aside, a mutation for survival cannot be present in only one person or even two people. Many people must possess it because the survivors of a highly lethal stress must produce the next generation and the parent population cannot be too small or too closely related.)

Do mutations for HIV resistance exist in the human population? Yes, at least one such gene for HIV resistance has already been identified.[54] Ideally, such a mutation would be a pre-existing gene and, even better, it would be several different mutations but for the same thing. For example, there are a number of sickle-cell and thalassemia mutations conveying some degree of resistance to malaria infection throughout Africa, the Mediterranean, and the Indian Ocean regions.

Second, there has to be an environmental stress that is sufficiently strong to favor those individuals with the mutation while eliminating those without it. Third, the rate of adaptation depends primarily on the length of a generation. That is, evolution depends on how quickly the parents with the genes for tolerating the stress can produce offspring that are also able to tolerate the stresses faced by the parents.

One common estimate of the time necessary for adaptation of new traits in an entire population is 100 generations. This is the rub. For humans with a generation time of about 15-20 years, something on the order of 1000-2000 years might be needed for an adaptation to become common throughout the population. There are some ways to speed up the rate of adaptation, but those alternatives are not pleasant ones because…

As I mentioned previously, it is important to note that, as a species, population, or culture, we really do not *want* to adapt. Not at all. Adapting is not fun. The requirement of having stress in the environment that is strong enough to cause genetic change in a population has a rather critical requirement attached to it. That requirement is this: *most of the population has to die in a relatively short period of time,* and the stress has to exist for several generations to eliminate the weak genotypes and to favor the strong ones to the point that they dominate the gene pool. That is, *adaptation requires*

---

[54] An interesting article on this mutation: Zrinka Biloglav, et al. 2009. Historic, Demographic, and Genetic Evidence for Increased Population Frequencies of CCR5Δ32 Mutation in Croatian Island Isolates after Lethal 15th Century Epidemics. *Croatian Medical Journal* 50:34-42. And incidentally, the CCR5-Δ32 allele was the focus of the attempt by Chinese researcher He Jiankui to create HIV resistant children in 2018.

death, a lot of it, and for a long time. If the death rate is lower, the time for adaptation is longer; for adaptation to occur quickly, the death rate must be extremely high.

As a population experiences such an intense stress, the death rate would likely be highest among the elderly but, unfortunately, for rapid adaptation to occur, it is far more important for the juveniles and the younger adults in the population to experience high mortality rates. For adaptation to occur in any species, the individuals without the necessary protective genes would be removed from the population, and *that must happen before those individuals can reproduce* and pass on their weaker (non-adaptive) genes. That means mortality must occur prior to adulthood, which can either mean before reproductive maturity or that reproduction itself would fail.

The death of adults who have already produced offspring does not affect the makeup of the population in a meaningful way because those adults have already passed on their genes. Only the death of their offspring *before* they have a chance to produce their own offspring matters in the course of adaptation. Those individuals with the mutation for resistance to the stress are the survivors and the successful reproducers. Their offspring will repopulate the depleted population.

Over the course of many generations, only those exhibiting resistance to an environmental stress, such as a lethal pathogen, will survive in the population. That population has now adapted to the stress, but it took several, perhaps many, traumatic generations. So, in short, humans are slow to adapt, and, in fact, we will do anything to avoid it.

If we think about what sorts of organisms adapt quickly, we should think of small, rapidly reproducing sorts of things. Let's use the generic term "bugs." Bugs, from bacteria to houseflies to cockroaches, can produce prodigious numbers of offspring in a short amount of time, and those offspring can produce their own offspring shortly after that.

For many, if not most small things, a large number of generations can elapse during the period of the stress, and that results in quick adaptation to the stress. For example, humans can apply a stress to a bug's environment over the course of a single year, but a year is an enormous amount of time for bugs. A year is often longer than the lifespan for many small things. For houseflies, a new generation can be produced in about two weeks, and one female fly can lay up to 500 eggs. At that rate, a pair of flies could produce 100 million million

(1.9×10^{14}) offspring *in a single summer* if all offspring survived long enough to reproduce.

If a sufficiently intense stress were present, such as an insecticide that quickly and effectively eliminated non-resistant flies, this rate of reproduction meets all the requirements for rapid adaptation. If a few insecticide-resistant individuals are present in the large fly population, the offspring of those individuals will generate a resistant population very quickly. It would be a small population initially, but with the capacity to grow rapidly. In general, organisms that behave in this manner and can adapt rapidly to new stresses we can refer to as BUGS.

In contrast, "Big" species like humans, cats, and sharks, cannot quickly adapt to lethal environmental stresses because the period of intense stress is typically *much shorter than the amount of time needed* for producing new and adapted generations. That is, in a highly stressful environment, the individuals die quickly and before each new generation can grow old enough to produce their offspring.

For example, a pandemic such as the Spanish Flu of 1918 killed at least 50 million people worldwide but was already waning only six weeks after the main outbreak began. The stress was gone in a short amount of time relative to the generation time of humans. (The death toll was about 2.5% of the world population which is not sufficient to bring about a significant shift in global human genetics. Similarly, COVID-19 will also not result in a shift in human genetics.)

If a mutation exists in the population that confers resistance to the epidemic, those with the mutation will survive at much higher rates, but there are some additional difficulties. First, the resistant survivors would have to be of reproductive age, not too young and not too old, to begin rebuilding the population. Second, the resistant survivors would have to mate and produce resistant offspring and (for humans) that process takes about a year.

Third, the resistant offspring require about 15 years to produce offspring of their own. The population would recover much too slowly. Perhaps more importantly, the stress that caused the increase in mortality would have long since faded from the environment, as with the Spanish Flu example. The mutation for resistance would be of no particular use unless the lethal stress returned repeatedly and was always deadly.

While the human species harbors a large number of random mutations (one estimate has it at about six per person), "random" implies that the vast majority of mutations will be of little use in a flu epidemic. And human populations within a particular region that might be affected by a specific stress are typically rather small populations compared to those of BUGS.

In contrast, BUG populations tend to be large and are likely to harbor a large number of mutations, many of which may be appropriate for tolerating new stresses. If a severe stress eliminates a large proportion of a large population of BUGS, the survivors are still numerous and capable of rebuilding the population quickly. In other words, in environments where short-lived and intense stresses occur (such as diseases), BUGS can adapt easily, and BIGS cannot.

So, if adapting takes so long, how did all of the BIGS in the world (especially humans) manage to stay alive for millions of years? Let's accept as a truism that no living species has ever faced a stress that was too intense to be accommodated through adaptation. Of course, that's circular reasoning; if a species exists, then it must have tolerated all stresses it faced through history because otherwise, it wouldn't exist. And that isn't an entirely correct statement either; species are made up of locally adapted and widely distributed populations, and it is common for a population to succumb to a local stress, but this does not mean the entire species disappeared.

However, most stresses that arise in an environment are not so lethal that every individual dies before the population is able to adapt to the stress. If we assume that any species (ourselves included) is faced with literally dozens of different environmental stresses that potentially can lower the life expectancy of different individuals in different ways but which don't kill outright, then we see that most stresses are not wiping out huge proportions of the populations. Those populations have longer periods of time to adjust and adapt to those different stresses. Thus, all BIGS have adapted throughout their history, but only to relatively low-intensity stresses or to stresses that did not affect the entire species simultaneously.

Chapter 15

Of BIGs And BUGs: Why The Little Things Matter

So again, how did all the BIGS in the world adapt if it takes so long for them? *Genetic change in a population is not the only way to survive stress*. The ability to make quick physiological adjustments is also an adaptation and does not require genetic change in the population every time stress occurs. If one is able to adjust quickly to changes in the environment, then the need for rapid genetic change is not as great.

For example, humans who move to high-altitude locations will quickly experience an increased number of red blood cells in their blood. It does not take years or generations. This is a physiological response to living in low oxygen environments and is one of a great many physiological adjustments humans can make to maintain our internal homeostasis. As "warm-blooded" creatures, we must maintain a relatively constant internal environment no matter what the external environment may be, and our physiological flexibility is absolutely key to that.

Our ability to make these changes is a genetic trait for rapid physiological adjustment; there is no need for our circulatory system to genetically adapt to life in the mountains. Humans are quite flexible in this way, and we are able to live in and adjust to a wide variety of environments. This flexibility is common to most species (especially plants) and we refer to the trait as *phenotypic plasticity*. It is the ability to change one's physiological and sometimes physical status, whether internal or external, in response to the conditions one experiences.

A well-known plant example of phenotypic plasticity is seen in the common ornamental Hydrangea bush. When growing in acidic soil (low pH), the flowers are blue, but when in neutral to basic soil (high pH), the flowers are pink. *The feedback from the external conditions changes the internal conditions* and this is reflected in the appearance of the flowers.

There might be no genetic difference between a pink bush and a blue bush, just a difference in the quality of the soil where the two plants are growing. And if a plant with blue flowers in low pH soil is transplanted to a higher pH soil, it will begin to produce pink flowers. (This, of course, is a source of frustration to gardeners who intentionally buy blue Hydrangeas but begin to get pink flowers after the plants have been in the new garden soil for a while.)

This plasticity allows organisms to adjust quickly to changing conditions. By adjusting to better tolerate the conditions, plasticity can help an organism buy the time necessary for adapting to a stress. If a biochemical adjustment reduces the effects of stress long enough for the individual to reproduce, then that ability has the appearance of an adaptation but is really the ability to make adjustments (which is also an adaptation).

If the stress is present over a long period of time, those individuals able to make such adjustments will come to dominate the population. Fine-tuning of the genetic ability will be favored in each generation, and the negative effect of the stress will steadily decrease. The population will have changed genetically, and therefore it adapted, but the adaptation is for the ability to alleviate the stress by making quick physiological adjustments.

Plasticity is an efficient mechanism for responding to changes in the environment. It's genetically based but relies on environmental cues to trigger the appropriate response. These cues might be changes in temperature, day length, humidity, food quality, or even soil pH. In fact, all organisms depend on environmental cues for a tremendous variety of growth, reproductive, and behavioral processes.

For example, zookeepers that tend flocks of flamingoes know that little if any mating and egg-laying will take place unless there is a threshold number of birds. That is, flamingoes rely on visual cues related to group size to stimulate the behaviors that lead to successful mating. Once the females are surrounded by a sufficient number of neighbors, the females are stimulated to begin the mating and nest-building processes. The minimum number of birds ranges from 14 to about 40, depending on the flamingo species. By synchronizing the mating and egg-laying among all females, the chicks are born simultaneously. In principle, the larger numbers of chicks reduce predation risk for each individual because the probability of being killed by a predator goes down when there is a larger number of chicks for the predator to choose from.

In plants, flowering is often tied to the length of the periods of light and dark, that is, the length of the day and night. Some plants flower as the nights get shorter (and the days longer), and some flower as the nights get longer (and the days shorter). In our gardens, these plants flower predictably at the same time each year. So how is it that we can go to the market or florist and buy flowers out of season?

The horticultural world manipulates the flowering in the plants by using greenhouses to change the length of the night period. Summer flowering plants will flower in the spring if the lights in the greenhouse are kept on for longer periods of time; spring flowers can be produced in the fall by turning on the lights at night to make the nighttime seem shorter. The plants respond to the light and dark periods and not to the time of year. These are genetically fixed responses to light and dark, but plants also demonstrate a wide variety of plastic responses to other environmental cues. Another obvious flowering response is to temperature. Unseasonably warm early spring weather will result in the early flowering of fruit trees.

Some plastic responses become stronger over time as sequential triggers cause the physiological response to become stronger with each episode. One obvious example in humans is the release of histamines triggered by pollen and the subsequent allergic reaction. Many allergy sufferers know that the response can become more and more emphatic with continued exposure to the environmental trigger. These responses are essentially defensive as the body is reacting to foreign proteins, and it attempts to eliminate or neutralize those proteins once they have entered our bodies. Many serious allergies are an ever-increasing over-reaction to the foreign molecules, and this is brought on by repetitive triggers from the environment. However, allergic responses may also be useful for defending the body from invasion by foreign proteins and microbes.

Genetically-based defenses require a trigger, a response, and deployment of the response to affected areas. However, acquiring new defenses (new adaptations) is still dependent on generation time and is not realistic for dealing with novel challenges from the environment. As BIGS, we are certainly capable of handling environmental stresses from our evolutionary past, but *how do we acquire new capacity to respond to new stresses,* and how do we do that in a reasonably short amount of time?

I suggest that human evolutionary history has favored a strategy for survival that is related to the food we eat. As Michael Pollan elegantly explained[55], humans are faced with interesting problems by being omnivores. Carnivores and herbivores do not share our problems because they eat one kind of food: mostly proteins or mostly plant materials, and the herbivores are often specific in their preferences. The digestive systems are less complex, chemically speaking, in comparison.

In contrast, an omnivore's digestive system must be flexible and able to tolerate and manage a wide variety of food types. That plasticity does not come easily because the ability to digest is a biochemical ability; an omnivore's digestive system must be able to produce a range of digestive enzymes and manage a wide range of food quality. The range of food quantity and quality may change daily, monthly, and seasonally. For example, a traditional human diet may follow a sequence where winter greens are replaced by spring root vegetables followed by summer fruits and grains. These are rather different types of foods with different digestive requirements. How did BIGS like us adapt to be able to eat such a variety of foods? Perhaps, we didn't have to.

BUGS adapt in very short amounts of time. Bacteria, in particular, are the most adept at shifting rapidly to accommodate change (as we noted earlier), and every human maintains trillions of these little fast-responders. With a microbiome numbering in the tens of trillions with hundreds to thousands of species, perhaps humans and other BIGS have a stimulus-reaction system already in place. If our microbiota can respond to the food we eat within a few hours, the microbiome could act as the rapid-response system we need.

We already know that BUGS can evolve faster than BIGS. Modifying the genetic architecture of a BIG takes many generations, measured in years, but changes in food quality happen over months and weeks, and even days. Unless we possess a large number of genes for producing a wide array of enzymes for digesting food of unpredictable quality (we don't) and those genes can be turned on and off easily (probably not), it is possible that the possession of a diverse microbiome reduces and even eliminates that need.

---

[55] Michael Pollan. 2006. *The Omnivore's Dilemma*. Penguin Press.

And as previously discussed, genetic responses to changes in the environment are hampered by the requirement of having appropriate mutations already present in the population, but such mutations are random. Random and chance processes in small populations (which is typical of humans throughout history) are inefficient for developing rapid and directed responses to stress. *Forming symbiotic associations with BUGS may have become an evolutionary answer for all BIGS to the problem of rapid response to environmental change* or of long-term response to environmental stresses for which there are no available mutations.

The diversity of the digestive microbiome in an omnivore and its ability to further diversify quickly represents an ideal mechanism for living in unpredictable, variable, diverse, and hazardous environments. Survival in such environments depends on adjusting and adapting to stress relatively quickly.

While BUGS are small and vulnerable to physical threats, they can manage the evolutionary process faster and more efficiently than BIGS, which are at a distinct disadvantage in that regard. We should not be surprised that symbiotic relationships between small and large organisms are common and are likely a requirement for survival as a BIG. The rapid evolutionary response of the BUGS and the physical hardiness of the BIGS is an ecological combination that provides an ideal arrangement for meeting the challenges of a shifting and unpredictable environment.

We Need No Stinkin' Adaptations

The original question at the top of Chapter 14 of whether we humans are adapting to our world should probably be answered with, "No, but we might not need to." We have BUGS on our side. Without a doubt, our systems do need to respond to environmental triggers that indicate stress, but our first response system in some, maybe many, cases is being managed by symbiotic microbes that can handle chores that are outside of our genetic capacity.

One estimate of the genetic diversity of the digestive microbiome is five million genes (and that may be on the low side). That is, our microbiome has 5,000,000 genes representing an incredible diversity of biochemical processes. In comparison, the Human Genome Project identified a paltry 20,000 genes in humans. In other words, we have a small base from which to draw when it comes to potentially useful mutations and it takes us years, nay decades, to produce more of them.

Again, this is not to say we don't have a long history of adapting to the environment, but that history is fraught with examples of how uncertain the process of adaptation can be. The period of 1347-1351 in Europe and the Mediterranean Basin is perhaps the most famous historical example of the human race being faced with an environmental challenge. Over the course of five years, the Bubonic Plague took an estimated 25-50 million lives representing about 40-60% of the region's population.[56] While it's hard to know the exact numbers, the consequences of losing nearly half the total population probably had a significant effect on the genetic make-up of the region.

Did the human population adapt? No, not overall, because 40% mortality is not strong enough to cause a rapid adaptive shift in the population. However, in some areas, entire villages were lost, and in those areas, the effects of the plague might be noticeable. The Plague returned many times over the subsequent 150 years, but if the necessary evolutionary requirement of genetic variation is not met (that is, there are no mutations for genetic resistance), then there is no possibility of the survivors of the plague being anything other than lucky or hardy.

However, in Scandinavian countries, it appears there was a mutated gene (CCR5-Δ32) that conferred resistance to infection and that mutation remains relatively common in some areas to this day.[57] It is likely the carriers of the gene survived the onslaught of the plague and produced the majority of the offspring for several generations. The result is a regional population that is more resistant to plague than other areas of Europe despite the fact that all of Europe and the Mediterranean felt the ravages of the disease.[58]

The necessity of high mortality for genetic adaptation is unavoidable, but absolute numbers are not the same as relative numbers. The Spanish Flu pandemic of 1918 killed at least 50 million

---

[56] Estimates range as high as 200 million, but 28-50 million is more likely. William H. McNeill. 1976. *Plagues and Peoples*. Anchor/Doubleday. Sephanie Haensch, et al. 2010. Distinct clones of *Yersinia pestis* caused the black death. *PLoS pathogens*, 6(10), p.e1001134.

[57] S. R. Duncan, S. Scott and C. J. Duncan. 2005. Reappraisal of the historical selective pressures for the CCR5-Δ32 mutation. *Journal of Medical Genetics*, 42(3), pp.205-208.

[58] This is the same mutation that confers resistance to HIV infection noted earlier. This is linked to the fact that both Bubonic Plague and HIV attack the immune system through the T-helper cells. The similarities are remarkable because Plague is caused by a bacterium and HIV is a virus.

and perhaps as many as 100 million people worldwide, making it the worst epidemic in history in terms of the number of people killed. However, with a world population of about 1.9 billion, mortality was about 2.5-5.0% compared to the 40% mortality of the Bubonic Plague in Europe (and many other epidemics in that region). Consequently, the effects of what appears to be a devastating stress are imprinted in some populations but not in the genetic architecture of our species as a whole.

Technology To The Rescue?

With the rise of public vaccinations as a common medical procedure, starting about 1900, first for diphtheria and then for many others in rapid succession, the era of modern medicine began. At this point, the human species was able to protect itself from the many dangerous pathogens in our environment that had regularly taken a toll, especially on children. Prior to 1900, about 25% of children died before the age of two, and another 25% died during the toddler to teenage years.

Because of high child mortality, life expectancy was 40-50 years in 1900 (often much lower in less developed countries) and had been for a long time. If there had been a steady pressure on humans to adapt to these diseases, that pressure was eliminated by vaccines and later antibiotics. In a short time, the western world made the transition from being a world of infectious diseases to one dominated by age-related diseases (notably, cardiovascular diseases and cancers). This also represents a transition from death before reproduction to death after reproduction, and this meant *the era of potentially adapting to our environment was probably over*.

Chapter 16

E = MB2 Or We Need More Genes!

An organism's genome contains all of the information necessary to produce a mature reproductive adult from a single fertilized cell. One of the most fascinating aspects of genetics is that every non-reproductive cell in your body that possesses DNA also possesses the entire genome. However, each cell has a specific purpose and uses only the tiniest fraction of the available genetic information. The thousands of different kinds of cells in our bodies use different fractions of the genome, but the entire genome is probably used in one way or another at some time in our lives.

In that sense, the genome is like a vast library full of books and each person visiting the library is checking out different books on different subjects. No one has time to read the entire library, nor would doing so be of any particular value. When we go to the library, we typically want a specific portion of the information for a specific purpose. That's essentially what the cells in our bodies do with the vast amount of information in the human genome.

Of course, when we were embryos, each embryonic cell was undifferentiated and it produced a lineage of trillions of cells that each would eventually have a particular vocation. While the embryonic cell was using very little of the genetic information, it would go on to produce a huge variety of cells that collectively were going to use a large portion of the genomic information. With each subsequent cell division and overall growth of the embryo, the resulting cells began to follow certain pathways and differentiate into particular cell types. As they did so, less and less of the available genetic information was relevant to the pathway they were on.

Eventually, as each tissue and organ formed, the cells developed specific functions and had access only to specific portions of the genetic code. A carpenter does not need a syringe; a nurse does not need a hammer. Skin tissue does not need to rhythmically contract; heart tissue does not need to sense touch. Nonetheless, all cells may interact either directly or indirectly with many other and different cells as part of their normal function.

Given our physical and biochemical complexity, the human genome has surprisingly few genes, about 20,000, on our 23 pairs of chromosomes. Every one of us has exactly the same genes in the same places on the same chromosomes. What makes us different are the versions of the genes, the *alleles*, that each of us possesses that together make each of us into distinct individuals. And because we have two copies of each chromosome, one from our mother and one from our father, the combination of the two alleles can create additional variation. We can express one allele or the other or both simultaneously. And we often have multiple genes for particular traits, like eye color, that add even more potential for variation. However, in many ways, it isn't the genes or the alleles of the genes that are interesting; it's the timing and intensity of the expression of the alleles and their interactions that can be mysterious.

The expression of a gene concerns the product that the gene codes for. For many years, geneticists thought that the phrase "one gene, one protein" reflected the way the cell decoded a gene to produce a protein and the role the protein played in the cell. That is, each gene is translated to produce a protein and that protein has a single job in the cell. The protein might be an enzyme that catalyzes a reaction, or it might be a building block as the cell produces new structures.

It was recognized that the long string of amino acids that formed each protein would curl and fold to form a three-dimensional structure, and that fixed shape was the activated protein. We now understand this is only true for some proteins and most proteins are much more complicated than that. For example, the biochemical conditions in the cell where the protein is being produced can determine how the amino acid string folds, and different 3-D conformations *of the same string of amino acids* will result in enzymes with different metabolic functions. Or an enzyme may have more than one binding site and, therefore, more than one function. Or, after performing one function, the shape of the enzyme can change to allow for a different function.

Enzymes can even split in two, with each fragment taking on a new capacity. The mystery behind enzymatic proteins and their functions is the timing of when, where, how, and on what other molecules are they acting. Enzymes can even influence the decoding and the expression of other DNA. That is, the magnitude of the expression of a gene can be influenced by not only the presence but the abundance of other proteins.

The oxygen-carrying molecule in our red blood cells is hemoglobin and is an example of alleles and the proteins they produce being turned on and turned off. Before we were born and still *in utero*, our bodies obtained oxygen from our mother's blood. The mother's blood doesn't mix with the baby's blood because the two are in separate circulatory systems, but the blood vessels in the placenta pass so closely that oxygen from the mother's blood diffuses into the baby's blood.

This indirect access to oxygen works because the embryonic blood of the fetus has a higher affinity for oxygen than the adult blood of the mother, and the oxygen moves easily from her system to the fetus. Our blood is made up of small red blood cells that contain hemoglobin molecules, which is a complex molecule made up of four subunits of two different globin molecules. Embryonic blood is not the same as the mother's blood: the maturing embryo produces blood subunits made of two molecules, each of alpha and gamma globins and the mother's adult blood is comprised of alpha and beta globins.[59]

Just before a baby is born, the composition of the hemoglobin begins to shift from embryonic to adult globins over the course of several months. In other words, the gene for the gamma-globin protein is turned off (down-regulated), and the gene for the alpha-globin protein is turned on (up-regulated), and this is somehow facilitated by changes in the physical and biochemical environment of the fetus.

This is just one way the expression of our genes changes as the environment changes, no matter whether the "environment" is in the cell, in the organ, or external to the body. The expression of the genes depends on the environment in which the genes are being used; the effect of the environment can be to turn them off or on or to moderate

---

[59] The alpha and beta globins are 3-dimensional proteins that form a complex structure around an iron molecule. The iron molecule binds to oxygen and this is how oxygen is transported through the body. One red blood cell contains about 250 million hemoglobin units and an adult circulatory system may contain 25 trillion red blood cells.

their expression. *Thus, the phenotype of an organism depends on the environmental stimuli that affect the genome.*

For example, plants will produce defensive chemicals after they have been attacked by an herbivore. After detecting the presence of a predator, water fleas (*Daphnia*) will produce sharply pointed defensive structures on their shells and tadpoles will develop more muscular tails. In humans, defensive antigens aren't produced until after we are infected with a virus. The full development of our digestive system doesn't occur until after we are exposed to and colonized by certain bacteria in our gut. It all comes AFTER because these changes represent *responses to the environment.*

Our Phenotype is the result of the interaction between the Genotype and the Environment, which is to say that our physical and physiological status depends on how our genetics are stimulated by the environment. (Evolutionary biologists abbreviate this interaction: $P = G \times E$.) The constantly changing external world of living and nonliving factors forces our biological systems to react, to adjust, and to compensate in order to maintain a stable internal environment. And we *must* maintain a stable internal environment.

The homeostasis of our internal environment is critical to efficient functioning and is tightly regulated by many feedback systems that track inputs and stimuli and then respond accordingly. If we get too hot, we sweat, and the evaporation of the sweat cools us. If we become dehydrated and our blood becomes more concentrated, we are stimulated to drink. These are our physiological reactions to the consequences of being in our environment.

We also interact with the living components of our external environment and some of those interactions are close and intimate. Hundreds of species of bacteria and larger organisms live in the dozens of different locations and niches on our skin. Hundreds more species live in our mouth. Some species don't live on us so much as we live near them and amongst them in our clothes and in our homes. We know little about important interactions that may exist between those organisms and our biology, particularly with regard to the health of our skin and our oral, nasal, otic, vaginal, and anal cavities and orifices. And what we are now coming to understand is that our "environment" is not just the external world but the internal world too, and sometimes it's hard to tell the difference.

The microbiota within us helps to regulate and maintain our internal environment. At the very least, the digestive microbiome controls the rate at which food materials move through us. In a broader sense, however, the internal microbiome filters and manages inputs from the external environment, whether in the form of food materials or other microbial introductions. This filtering process is one that, for the most part, we lack as humans. Left to ourselves, it is unlikely our system could manage all that enters our bodies through our mouths as efficiently as we do with the help of our microbiome.

To a pathogenic bacterium, our bodies are a rich and untapped resource with a few antibiotic defenses, and any bacterium that overcomes those defenses will have won the bacterial sweepstakes. However, our microbiome is comprised of thousands of other species of bacteria that will compete for resources, dominate the different niches, and actively resist the colonization of other newly-arriving species, whether they are pathogenic or not.

Under normal conditions, a healthy ecosystem is diverse, stable, resistant to change, and resilient in the face of change. This complexity acts as an incredibly strong filter preventing colonization by new bacteria. Dozens to hundreds of bacterial species attack the food materials moving through our intestine, and they probably leave little available space for newcomers.[60] The mucosal lining of the intestine is densely packed with colonies of many species that are finely adapted to the conditions there; few newly-arriving species can gain a foothold.

The environmental conditions, from the entry to the large intestine at the cecum all the way to the exit at the anal sphincter, vary tremendously[61], and each section of the colon is filled with bacteria that are well suited to those conditions. New bacterial introductions to the existing microbiome will go through an extensive vetting process; a new colonist would have to be tolerant of the acidic environment of the stomach, resistant to the antimicrobial environment of the small intestine, and then be highly competitive for space on the intestinal lining or highly competitive for the food material moving through the colon.

In short, the environmental stimuli that result in the phenotype may be more correctly understood as *the interaction of the two microbiomes* that directly and indirectly stimulate the expression of

---

[60] And obviously, the opposite is also true. People with very simplified microbiomes will be much less resistant to invasion and colonization by new microbes. And this implies that such individuals will be more prone to new and recurrent diseases.

[61] Gregory P. Donaldson, A. Melanie Lee, Sarkis K. Mazmanian. 2016. Gut biogeography of the bacterial microbiota. *Nature Reviews: Microbiology* 14:20-32

the genotype. We are just now expanding our appreciation of the contribution of the internal microbiome to the intricacies of homeostasis of the human body. There is no question that the microbiome stimulates and helps develop the immune system, that it provides necessary nutrients to our bodies, that it defends us from pathogenic bacteria, and that it influences our physical and physiological development. There is also no question that our microbiome cannot survive without the human body providing a suitable habitat. It is a true mutualistic relationship except that the microbiome is an entire community of a thousand or more species, and they fill many different niches in the habitat that we call our gut, and together the human body and the microbiome create a complex ecosystem.

We also know that the microbiome did not appear *de novo* in our digestive tract but has developed over our lifetimes from the sterile environment of the newborn to the complex, interactive, self-regulating ecosystem of the adult person. However, we know little about the assembly process and rates of colonization.

We know the first bacteria to enter the digestive system of the newborn are oral, vaginal, and anal bacteria of the mother, plus additional important bacteria from her breast milk. Those bacteria begin the process of colonization of the digestive system, they aid in the breakdown of complex molecules, and their presence in the digestive tract facilitates further colonization by creating a low-oxygen environment that is more appropriate for other bacterial species.

The eventual "biogeography" of the digestive system results in oxygen-dependent species living toward the front end of the digestive tract and those favoring low-oxygen or no-oxygen environments occupying the back end of the digestive tract. Of course, this process of colonization is made more complex with the consumption of solid and slow-to-digest food as this becomes the primary resource for the later-arriving bacteria. These bacteria are introduced to the baby in different ways but from the external environment.

Obviously, the mother, father, and siblings in the household create a bacterial environment that introduces appropriate bacteria to the newborn. The baby's gut microbiome will strongly resemble those of the members of the household regardless of their genetic similarity. Other bacteria will be introduced through contact with other people, places, and things in the environment, including the food the growing child eats. This process of adding diversity will continue for several years and will be highly dynamic over the course of a lifetime.

Our understanding of the P = G x E equation has to be expanded to include an appreciation of the contribution of both the external microbial environment and the ever-increasing diversity and complexity of the internal microbiota. In terms of digestion, immunology, metabolism, and some developmental processes, we have to acknowledge that the environment we experience is greatly influenced by TWO microbiomes that interact with each other such that our Environment (E) is the interaction between MB $_{external}$ and MB $_{internal}$ or we can abbreviate that to E = MB^2 just to be clever.

The two ecosystems cannot be separated; the internal microbiome is highly dependent on the external system for inputs, but the external microbiome in the near vicinity of each person (e.g., the household) is also influenced by the internal microbiome.

Given the recent discoveries of the intense and intricate interactions between human physiology and the gut microbiome, *and* the dependence of the internal microbiome on colonization by the external microbiome, *and* the fact that these interactions begin at birth can continue until death, we are faced with the realization that we know less than we thought about how our bodies work *on their own*. The studies of germ-free laboratory animals have clearly shown abnormal intestinal development and altered immunological capacity in the absence of gut bacteria. The implications for humans are under intense investigation, but what isn't in doubt is the essential requirement of gut microbes for what we consider normal human development and health.[62]

If our genetic expression is dependent on the environment and the environment is made up of two interacting microbiomes, then as part of our quest for understanding our health, *we have to reconsider our personal orientation to the external world*. While the evidence is rapidly mounting that the internal microbiome is of unquestionable importance for internal homeostasis and health in humans, it will also become impossible to argue that the internal environment should be considered in any way separate or disconnected from the external environment.

---

[62] Felix Sommer and Fredrik Bäckhed. 2013. The gut microbiota – masters of host development and physiology. *Nature Reviews: Microbiology* 11:227-237.

Although the mature gut appears to have a diverse and stable microbiota and the appendix may act as an emergency reservoir,[63] the flux of bacteria from the external environment is likely to play an important role in keeping the internal microbiota up-to-date and relevant. While we do not have any estimates of rates of exchange between the two worlds, researchers are now turning their attention to the role of our food in supplying bacteria to the gut microbiome.[64]

---

[63] R. Randal Bollinger, et al. 2007. Biofilms in the large bowel suggest an apparent function of the human vermiform appendix. *Journal of Theoretical Biology* 249:826-831.

[64] In particular, the American Gut portion (led by Dr. Rob Knight) of the Human Food Project (led by Dr. Jeff Leach) seek to understand the influence of diet (and many other variables) on the microbiome. With a large enough dataset, it should be possible to find strong relationships between specific dietary choices and microbial diversity. While this doesn't measure microbe flux with the external environment, it will add tremendously to the very little we know about the dietary influences on the human microbiome.

Chapter 17

Here's The Rub:
BUGS Help BIGS Stay Relevant

From an evolutionary biology point of view, exchanges with the environment (or at least an inward movement) would provide valuable information to the microbiome about the external environment and could help to optimize digestive efficiency and responsiveness to new food material. The capacity of the microbiota to respond to new food materials is based on previous experience. That is, we have the genetic capacity to digest basic food components (simple carbohydrates, fats, protein), but as BIGs we do not have the capacity to respond rapidly to significant changes in our environment without help from the BUGs.

The microbiota is a large and diverse collection of BUGs with a vast genetic profile and rapid reproductive potential. The more species diverse the microbiota is and the more genetically diverse it is, the greater the potential for being able to manage new food materials and adjust to them in a relatively short period of time.

While BIGs cannot adapt rapidly and cannot easily adjust to environmental conditions with which they have no prior evolutionary experience (such as a novel source of food), the bacteria associated with that food or that same environment may be able to make rapid adjustments for us. Our evolutionary past, involving thousands of years of living in a particular region and eating the foods of that region, has molded our digestive ability and, in some cases, in specific ways.[65] It likely takes thousands of years for such adaptations in

---

[65] In *Food, Genes, and Culture* (2013, Island Press) Gary Paul Nabhan writes about the tight link between cultures and their foods and gives special attention to

humans to take place, and so it is also a survival imperative to have the capacity for rapid adjustment. Our microbiome provides that.

Humans have the genetic capacity for handling a range of food types, but there is no way to anticipate sudden changes or novel food materials, and the human system does not have unlimited capacity. Thus, most animals and especially all omnivores (such as ourselves) possess diverse microbiomes that can adjust to manage new food material. The possession of the microbiome is itself an adaptation because it keeps us alive, healthy, and reproductive. The more capable our microbiome is, the healthier we are. In a bacterial sense, being capable means being diverse and up-to-date with respect to the surrounding environment and to the stream of food materials moving into and through the body.

A bacterial community that is up-to-date and relevant is one that is regularly challenged by the environment and that, by necessity, means interactions between the internal and external worlds. *The movement of bacteria into our digestive microbiome from the external microbiome is the movement of environmental information.* New bacterial species and new genotypes of current species represent genetic information because those new colonists possess different genetic abilities.

If those genetic additions confer new traits, different responsiveness, or new digestive capacity, then the microbiome has greater capacity relative to the flow of food materials that are being consumed by the host organism. This, in turn, would accelerate responsiveness and shorten response time when new food materials are encountered in the large bowel and thereby lead to less digestive distress and more efficient digestion.

I think we have to assume that certain foods would facilitate this important and necessary flow of information to the microbiome. New food materials, with which we might need some digestive assistance, are almost certain to be indigestible plant materials and secondary plant compounds (because we are fully capable of managing basic fats, proteins, and carbohydrates). Ingesting uncooked meat carries a risk of introducing pathogenic bacteria, so the sources of additions to the microbiome probably are from plant materials.

---

the idea that not only did humans adapt over long periods to the foods of the ethnic region, but in some cases the foods are necessary for general health. Specifically, some types of foods that are not part of the culture may be unhealthy because there is no adaptive history with them.

Fresh fruits and vegetables would be a likely source of new colonists because cooking and processing plant materials would essentially sterilize the foods and eliminate microbes (except those associated with spoilage). We can predict that a diet of highly processed and easily digested foods would not assist in the flow of new information, just as we know that low fiber diets with little plant material will likely reduce microbial diversity in the gut.

In contrast, diets high in novel and unusual fresh plant material may create digestive difficulties because of a different balance of celluloses, chitins, lignins, pectins, and some kinds of starch. In addition, plants produce a huge variety of toxins to discourage herbivory in the form of phenols, alkaloids, and terpenes. These compounds are particularly important because many of them have antibacterial qualities or interfere with chemical breakdown by microbes. An inexperienced digestive tract may lack the microbial diversity necessary to adjust to such new foods, but because humans do eat a tremendous variety of plant types around the world, we can safely predict that gut microbes that specialize on or are tolerant of these plants do exist.

If the microbiome does not receive regular information and maintain high genetic diversity, its resilience in the face of change may be compromised.[66] Ecological research strongly suggests that less diverse systems are less resilient, but we should also expect that out-of-date and isolated systems are less resilient too. For example, a person on a specific and low diversity diet is not actively challenging the digestive microbiome and can potentially lose diversity, especially with periodic flushing of the system due to diarrhea events or antibiotic use.

A digestive system with lower diversity will be less resilient and potentially less resistant to pathogenic colonizers and, therefore, more prone to disease. Indeed, the increasing frequency of stubborn *Clostridium difficile* (C-diff) infections is directly related to the use of antibiotics that reduce species diversity and invasion resistance in the gut. These conditions invite opportunistic infections and dominance.

In summary, given what we know and are learning about the importance of a healthy and stable internal microbiome to our health,

---

[66] An imperfect analogy is that of virus protection on your computer. When virus protection is out of date, the computer is naïve relative to external threats. Updated virus protection is essentially new information about the outside world that protects the computer from invasion and damage.

we must predict that such stability is based on ecological and evolutionary principles, as are all other processes governing living things. An important part of that stability is active, vital, and frequent exchanges between ecosystems. We should certainly expect the discovery of interesting nuances concerning these ecosystem interactions, but the vitality of the internal ecosystem will be predictably dependent to some degree on the vitality of the external ecosystem.

Whether this dependence is a long-term function or also has short-term aspects, and whether that changes over one's lifetime, will be a fascinating avenue of research. Given the importance of the microbiome to the human system, we know that this symbiotic interaction has existed for millions of years, and the stability of the microbiome, its ability to recover quickly, its close relationship with our physiology, and its dependence on our internal environment all reflect an evolutionarily significant link to our ability to survive.

Basically, we are probably protected from short-term fluctuations in the environment because of our microbiome, but the microbiome is also reliant on a flow of information from the environment for its and our long-term health.

Based on principles and evidence, I think we must conclude that the health of our personal ecosystem depends in a very real way on the health of the external ecosystem. Damage to the internal microbiome has an effect on our health and we are just beginning to realize the implications. But perhaps just as important is that damage to the external ecosystem, particularly to the external microbiome, will have an effect on the internal microbiome because of the loss of potentially important genetic information. The destruction or simplification of our ecosystems, or the loss of ecosystem components, may well have ramifications that we can't anticipate specifically but which we can predict generally.

By simplifying our external world, we are losing genetic information in the form of microbial species that may be necessary for our long-term health. Just as losing one or a few species from a diverse ecosystem may not have obvious dramatic effects because there are additional species to fill the roles of the lost species, the repeated loss of species will eventually result in loss of ecological functions when no species remain to fill certain niches. Such losses result in wholesale shifts in the attributes of the ecosystem. Some of those losses may not be tolerable.

Part III

The Owner's Manual
(What You Can Do)

Chapter 18

The Good, The Bad, And The Context Is Everything

Good Bacteria Vs. Bad Bacteria?

To put it plainly, in our everyday life, there is no such thing as good bacteria or bad bacteria. This may fly in the face of everything you've ever heard or read about bacteria, but it's true. No matter what we think of *Streptococcus* after several bouts of strep throat or *Staphylococcus* after a serious post-operative infection, those bacteria are only pathogenic under certain circumstances and usually when something has affected our ability to control their growth. Our deep-seated fear of bacteria is based on centuries of battling and dying from bacterial infections, plagues, and epidemics, but that fear represents a narrow view of the bacterial world.

Bacteria are everywhere. The ocean can be considered a bacterial soup with perhaps 20 billion bacterial cells per cubic meter in open ocean water. That's a large number, to be sure, but not particularly high population density for something as small as a bacterium, which is typically $1/100^{th}$ the length of a human cell. Nonetheless, there's a lot of ocean out there.

Bacteria are also incredibly abundant in natural soils and have been estimated at 10 billion per gram of soil with perhaps 1000 different kinds. The much higher numbers in soil compared to water is partly because there is a substrate (soil particles) for the bacteria to cling to and food is abundant. Nonetheless, we can assume that bacteria are present wherever there are molecules for them to consume.

The biggest problem for microbiologists is determining just what a bacterium species is, which seems like an odd problem. Bacteria are just about the simplest organisms you can imagine. One cell, no visible structures in the cell, and their food sources are organic materials they find in the environment. If there are organic molecules somewhere in the environment, there are bacteria trying to eat them.

Each type of bacteria has a particular food preference, some type of chemical that they are especially good at breaking down for energy, and when they find that food, they proliferate. Because there are few visible identifying characteristics and an individual bacterium is so small, it is hard to determine what species a bacterium might be. So, it's necessary to grow a colony of bacteria of a particular type and then test them in one of two ways: offer them a variety of food sources to see which ones they eat or obtain their genetic sequence. Both techniques then require a computer-assisted search that matches the food preferences or genetic profile to a particular species.

To further complicate the identification of a bacterial species, bacteria mutate frequently, and eventually, that complicates proper identification. In fact, the computer-assisted identification typically brings back a report something like: "there is an XX% chance of this being Species Z." That is, the identification of a species is rarely 100% certain. So, it's common just to lump bacteria into family groups, such as "coliform bacteria," which means they resemble *E. coli*. (i.e., they are rod-shaped, Gram-negative, non-spore-forming bacteria that contain the enzyme B-galactosidase).

In the case of the microbiome, few bacteria are actually named but are just listed as being members of, for example, the Proteobacteria, Firmicutes, or Bacterioidetes. As far as we're concerned, we really just want to know what they eat and what they do. Mostly, bacteria chemically break down other molecules to get energy and nutrients. That is, they digest molecules.

They also are particularly good at defending themselves, which is probably more accurately stated as they are good at defending the food they are trying to digest. They do this chemically also. Production of those defense and digestive chemicals is how bacteria survive in a world of billions of other bacteria and fungi species, most of which are potential competitors.

The defense chemicals that bacteria produce can take many forms, but in the world of microbes, chemical warfare is the primary mode of interaction, and those chemicals often affect the cell membranes of other species. This is relevant to the human relationship with bacteria because whether the bacteria are beneficial or pathogenic, the chemicals are the way the bacteria interact with our cells.

Most humans have 1,000-1,500 species of bacteria in their large intestine and all of them are secreting chemicals into the colon environment. This is what bacteria do. The bacteria are attempting to obtain energy and nutrients from the undigested plant materials that make it through the small intestine and are destined for excretion.

Given a sufficiently diverse bacterial community and a diversity of food materials, no one bacterial species can dominate the environment, which is also changing daily with the arrival of new and different foodstuff. So, the many species wax and wane in abundance as favored food supplies appear and then disappear. The abundance of each bacterial type can only increase in the immediate vicinity of its food supply, and as that food supply moves through the colon to the anus, the majority of the associated bacteria are carried along with it. And so, any particular group of bacteria is being moved toward the exit relatively quickly (about 18-24 hours) and the interaction with the host is short-lived and pretty neutral.

So, what is a bad bacterium? Simply put, a bad bacterium is one that is allowed (for some reason) to proliferate unchecked. This happens when the controls that normally slow or stop proliferation are absent or damaged. It may be at the site of an injury where only a few types of bacteria establish and the defenses of the body are not strong enough to suppress that growth. It may be in the colon after antibiotics have ravaged the bacterial diversity and only antibiotic-resistant bacteria remain. Resistant bacteria tend to be those that have a long history with the antibiotics that are used to control their growth.

In other words, if the environmental context changes, the resistance and resilience of the environment (such as the one in your colon) is compromised, and any bacteria that can take advantage of that situation can rapidly become super-abundant. Again, this is what bacteria do naturally. As I said before, *C. diff, E. coli, Streptococcus,* and *Staphylococcus aureus* are commonly occurring bacteria in the large intestine and can be identified in virtually everyone's fecal samples. When they occur in a healthy context, they are not problematic. When the context changes, they can be deadly. And so, good, bad, or neutral completely depends on the context.

How did we arrive at this bacterial-human, hard-to-comprehend, Gordian-knot of a mess? It's best to remember that under healthy (i.e., normal) conditions, the bacteria within us are not only benign, but we are learning that many of them are absolutely necessary to our health.

Why are some better than others? Do we need all of them? First, let's revisit the roles that bacteria play in our internal ecosystem.

Chapter 19

Obligate Mutualisms: We're Inseparable Buddies

Obligate mutualisms are evidence of a long and beneficial history of interaction between two organisms, with one typically being "host" to the other. The association is so entrenched that the two cannot live separately under normal conditions, but that doesn't mean the solo situation can't happen.

For example, a serious environmental and global problem of today is coral bleaching. When corals experience certain stresses, they expel the mutualist photosynthetic algae (zooxanthellae) embedded in the coral tissue, and the tissue becomes transparent or "bleached." All of the color from the algae is lost, and the white of the coral skeleton becomes visible. Without the zooxanthellae to provide the corals with food in the form of carbohydrates (sugar) from photosynthesis, the corals will slowly starve unless the ocean waters are rich in small organisms that can be captured as food.

There are several reasons why the zooxanthellae are expelled from the coral, but all are environmental stresses such as abnormally-high water temperatures, pollution, pathogens, sedimentation, and wildly fluctuating environmental conditions. Without the algae in their tissues, corals are dependent on their own ability to capture food, which they are fully capable of doing, but tropical coral reef zones have a reputation for clear water, and this is precisely because of the low abundance of tiny living things. It's for this reason that the mutualism between corals and algae formed in the first place - as a mechanism for living in an otherwise ideal habitat that had low food supplies.

Humans are faced with similar problems. A rich and diverse digestive ecosystem is a healthy condition. Many species of bacteria have likely been associated with us for so long that they have assumed some of the functions that humans used to have, or they have provided functions that we didn't have but that were highly beneficial to us. At some point, the bacteria became indispensable.

The current understanding is that one role of the microbiome is to stimulate our immune system, and this may have been an evolving role for bacteria in the gut. In primitive systems, if a bacterium took up residence, the system would have to protect itself from the presence and possible negative effects of the bacterium. That is, a healthy system should respond to the presence of the bacterium and be stimulated to defend itself whenever the bacteria are detected, but not when the bacteria are not detected. In a long-lived organism with different life stages, the presence of certain bacteria could evolve to be the trigger indicating that "it's time" to produce defensive functions.

For example, a newborn infant has no defensive abilities, but the colonization of the colon by bacteria provided by the mother acts as a signal that the baby's protective functions should be activated or that further maturation or development of the immune system is necessary. In other words, if the development of our immune system is coincident with the colonization by certain bacteria in the colon, then it's likely that over a long period of time, *the presence of those bacteria has become a necessary signal* for our timely and normal development.

What if the bacteria that stimulate the development of the immune system never arrive or are killed off? Current research is strongly suggesting that underdeveloped immune systems may be a long-term consequence of the bacterial conditions we experience in infancy. If vaginal birth and breastfeeding provide the first contact with bacteria to the sterile body and digestive system of the infant, the earliest developmental pathways may be affected.

The development of the immune and digestive systems seems to be a rapid but drawn-out process; it begins early but doesn't happen overnight. The early inoculation of the baby's microbiome by the mother appears to be important, but a delay in that inoculation will not stop the systems from developing more or less normally. In contrast, preventing the colonization of beneficial bacteria for an extended period may prevent normal development during the appropriate window of opportunity.

And so, vaginal vs. cesarean birth, breast milk vs. formula, and the use of antibiotics at birth and during infancy are all linked to changes to physiological and even physical development as infants move through different growth stages. The key to understanding this damage lies in understanding exactly when some of the interactions between the baby and the new microbiome are occurring, but it is likely this is not an exact calculation and varies from one person to the next.

While obligate bacterial mutualists may be important for certain developmental processes in the human body and even for ongoing functions and processes, we also don't know much about our innate capacity in the absence of the microbiome. That is, if some important bacteria are missing, do we still have the genetic ability to perform the functions ourselves? If we receive the appropriate stimulus in some other way, can we form and perform the needed functions?

Research on the interaction between the microbiome and the immune system will help answer those and many more questions, but it is important to remember a few things: First, we are BIGS and the bacteria are BUGS. *They can respond to changes in the environment quickly and can draw on millions of genes that humans do not possess.* That doesn't prevent us from possessing and maintaining an ability for proper development when the bacteria are absent, but we have only 20,000 genes to draw from. However, it is certainly possible that the speed and efficiency of those functions may be impaired by long-term non-use (that is, over the previous hundreds of generations).

Second, *the environment changes constantly*. If there is a need for a new function or a need for an enhanced function, we will be unlikely to produce it ourselves. And it's also possible that new or enhanced functions might be needed at a range of intensities and not merely as an on/off switch. Our microbiome's genome is far better suited to handle such demands than our genome is. Given the millennia that the microbiome has been involved in our development, digestion, and immunity, it is possible that we never had the need to adapt to a changing environment in the traditional sense.

The fact that humans, as BIGS, are as physiological adjustable as we are, that we have expanded our population to cover the globe, and that we are as omnivorous as we are, suggests that we have ceded a great deal of our evolution to the BUGS that we are associated with. And in return, despite being BIGS, we gained the abilities of BUGS to respond rapidly to important and regular changes in the environment, such as seasonal changes in food quality and diseases.

Third, *any loss of obligate mutualists in our personal ecosystem must have a cost*. All recent research points to the microbiome as being a required component of childhood development and a healthy adult life. The loss of obligate bacteria will likely be directly related to loss of function, protection, stimulus, and capacity.

There is no doubt: *we are not individuals; we are ecosystems.* As ecosystems, we depend on diversity for stability, functionality, resilience, resistance, and in other ways. Losing obligate mutualists in our microbiome would be like losing a limb that cannot be regrown; it is something we should avoid.

Chapter 20

Facultative Mutualisms: We're Just Good Friends

The wide variety of foods we eat means that we ingest a wide variety of chemical substances. As mentioned before, plants possess hundreds of thousands of secondary metabolites, most of which are related to defense against herbivores and many of which present digestive challenges for us.

All of these chemicals are toxins of one sort or another and their toxicity to us will depend on the concentration in the plant tissues. It would be absurd to think that the human gut is capable of handling them all. For one, with our paltry 20,000 genes, we just don't have the capacity to deal with such a variety.

Perhaps more importantly, food moves through our small intestine in about 90 minutes, and all of our digestion and absorption must be accomplished in that amount of time. Obviously, we can handle simple digestive tasks in the form of proteins, fats, and simple carbohydrates, and the absorption of important vitamins and minerals. Chemically complex substances that are difficult to break down cannot be managed in 90 minutes and, in fact, might require more energy to digest than they actually provide.

Thus, adaptations for handling such foods never happened in our evolutionary history because it was unnecessary for our survival. And we are either unaffected by plant toxins or we stopped eating certain plants because of the toxic effects. So, when it comes to slow-to-digest substances, we digest what we can and the rest passes on to the colon and through our system. We certainly don't need bacteria to handle the food material that we can't digest; in an evolutionary sense, we don't really care if it gets digested or not. In fact, things that we can't digest easily are usually not even referred to as "food."

Nonetheless, although we possess a repository of undigested material in our large intestine that we as humans are unable to use, that certainly does not mean that material is unusable. As with every ecosystem, we expect that unused resources are soon discovered by organisms that can make use of them.

However, everything about our colon suggests that we have slowed down the movement of undigested food for some reason, but not because we need more time to digest it. If we don't need it and can't make use of it, why does it suddenly move so slowly after zipping through the small intestine? In comparison to the small intestine, the large intestine is less muscular and has much slower contractions, which leads to a retention time of up to 24 hours even though the colon is a much shorter organ.

This sudden hitting of the brakes when food material enters the colon does not suggest in any way that we are finished with this food because it's unusable, but rather that we are going to hold on to it for a while longer, much longer than would seem necessary. The only reason seems to be that the indigestible stuff helps us create an environment suitable for the microbiome.

The tremendous diversity of bacteria in the colon does not imply that all bacteria are necessary or even beneficial. This is a niche filled with food, and the many hundreds of species merely reflect the diversity of food material, not a diversity of beneficial mutualisms. It's certainly possible that the majority of the species are benign and merely opportunistically filling a niche.

All of the bacteria produce enzymes that break down durable, complex, structural components of the food we send to them. These enzymes form a chemical soup that breaks chemical bonds in the food molecules. This process releases energy and breaks off smaller molecules that can be easier for other bacteria to break down further. What may be the most important aspect of the process of digesting cellulose from plants is that each bacterial species has one or more genes for producing enzymes that humans cannot produce.

Thus, living in our gut is a community of tens of trillions of tiny cells that collectively possess millions of genes, and, in a sense, we have access to those genes or at least to the gene products. Between the basic life-history properties of BUGS and their tremendous range of biochemical capacity, we have access to a system that provides rapid responses using an arsenal of chemical weapons that we, as

BIGS, could never have evolved independently. By consuming our omnivore diet, we maintain this vast array of functions and abilities even if we don't need them every day or even every month.

In this sense, *bacterial diversity provides for human digestive flexibility*. For example, people who eat a wide variety of food types, including spices, have a much more diverse digestive microbiome than someone raised on a diet of processed white bread, fried chicken, and mashed potatoes and who never gets adventurous with food.

The high-diversity microbiome is better able to handle food challenges without gastric upset and flatulence. It can handle the new food quickly and with a minimum of fuss. The low-diversity microbiome handles the foods it knows well, but it might not be able to accommodate new food types. And adjusting to new foods may take longer and may not be possible. A good example of that inflexibility is frequently seen in people eating spicy food for the first time or, actually, anywhere from 3-24 hours *after* they eat that food.

The human ability to provide a safe harbor for ten thousand species of bacteria (and counting) means that even if most of them are just hitchhikers, their presence can act as a safety net in a dynamic world, a chemical insurance policy against unforeseen events. Just as some bacteria may be obligate mutualists and we must have them for normal development, it is possible that *a microbiome of facultative mutualists is just as necessary*, just as obligate in a sense, for humans to persist in an ever-changing world.

Each particular species of bacteria may not be absolutely necessary, but the possession of a diverse and healthy microbiome is absolutely necessary, regardless of the exact makeup of that community. In that sense, anything that interferes with the normal functioning of a microbiome would be a danger to human health.

Chapter 21

Maintaining Our Balance

Losing Our Mutualists Is Like Losing A Limb.
Mutualists either enhance, replace, or provide functions. We lose obligate mutualists at our peril because not having them means not having the function they provide and that loss should predictably be followed by disease. If obligate bacteria support our health and physiological functions, the loss of those bacteria cannot be good. Fortunately, it should be difficult to do this because the 100% elimination of any bacteria is almost impossible.

When we experience disease after damage to the microbiome, it is likely that the healthy microbe populations have crashed to low numbers and are struggling to recover. If the colon environment is damaged or disturbed and becomes dominated by bacteria that cause pathogenic conditions, those conditions may prevent the obligate and beneficial bacteria from re-establishing. Any such situation would also involve the reduction of a great many facultative bacteria.

Deciphering the exact consequences of such losses in terms of any subsequent diseases is difficult. The disease could result from the loss of the function provided by the obligate species, but also could be from or compounded by the loss of the diversity and stability provided by the facultative species.

In the modern era (the one dominated by modern medicine), the loss of obligate bacteria may be one of the root causes of a number of new, curious, and difficult-to-understand diseases. An obligate mutualist bacterium, by definition, provides a benefit to its partner species, and the loss of that mutualist is accompanied by a loss of a *necessary* function.

For us to fully appreciate that relationship, we must also appreciate the complexity of the relationship, and this is where certain aspects of modern medicine may have reached their limits. A mutualism is an evolutionary process and that means it is capable of changing and, in fact, may be capable of a range of expression. That is, the expression can be low, medium, or high, depending on the situation.

Medical interventions are technological and geared toward the replacement of known and simple functions and are predicated on a single level of expression. That is, a bioactive chemical (medicine) is designed to provide a missing function in a straightforward fashion. However, the focus is on replacing the exact function *as it is understood by medical science*.

The medicine cannot replace the range of benefits that have been lost, nor can it operate as a replacement for a complex interaction. A therapeutic medicine replaces something that we, as humans, have identified as a lost function, but we typically lack a complete understanding of the disease associated with that loss of function.

Importantly, if we have lost a biological interaction provided by a biological entity, such as a bacterium, and replaced it with a technological solution, such as a medicine, we may be interfering with the ability of the human body to re-establish the original mutualism or its associated (and unknown) benefits. *The artificial medicine may act to prevent the restoration of the natural process*. Whether or not this is always the case, the goal of medicine is typically curative and not restorative.

It is also worth remembering that medicines are rarely tailored to the patient in any real sense. This is a characteristic of the one-size-fits-all approach of technology and medicine. I can only wear a shoe of a certain size, but in truth, my feet change shape over the course of a day, and my shoes cannot adjust in response. And I buy certain brands of shoes because of the differences in comfort and fit, but other people are comfortable buying brands that I find uncomfortable.

As mentioned before, anti-inflammatory or anti-histamine medicines may eliminate or reduce discomfort, but they do not address the underlying issue or issues that caused the discomfort, nor do they account for body size, personal medical history, family history, genetics, and so on. In that sense, *nearly all drugs are "generic" in that they address a specific ailment in a general way* and without any specificity for each of us as individuals.

In stark contrast, an obligate mutualist, such as a species of bacteria inhabiting our colon and living on the plant materials we consume, has a vested interest in maintaining the health of the colon environment. Indeed, the ability of humans to consume the range of plant foods that we do is a testament to the workings of the microbiome on our behalf.

Although it is a bit of a "Which came first: the chicken or the egg?" situation, we eat to feed the microbiome, and the microbiome protects our ability to keep eating, and that is the essence of a mutualistic relationship. More importantly, as our environment changes (for example, from summer to winter), the microbiome is capable of shifting too. If we experience a shift in our physiological functions over the seasons, perhaps due to temperature, activity levels, and the food we eat, the microbiome will shift with us.

It does not do this with any sense of intention, but because we are shifting the food supply flowing through the colon and the bacterial ecosystem, there is a shifting in abundance as a response. We predict that this response is moderated by the feedback from the host in terms of host health. That is, a healthy shift in bacterial diversity and abundance should be reflected in the maintenance of the host's health.

The importance of this relationship with regard to modern medicine is that medicines cannot shift in response to changes in host physiology. Medicine is inert in that respect, while bacteria are dynamic. If the microbiome is acting as a mutualistic barometer, the changes in the host are matched by changes in the microbial diversity and abundance as changes occur in the external environment and in terms of host physiology.

This is fundamentally what biological systems do: feedback from the environment stimulates changes that maintain homeostasis and ultimately maintain the stability and health of the system.

Chapter 22

How We Damage The Microbiome

Scene: A medieval castle and the village within its walls are under siege. The ranks of the soldiers have been depleted by injuries. The villagers are weak from days with limited food supplies, and now water is low and being rationed. The castle guards are losing the ability to defend the gates, and they can't maintain the strength of the fortifications. The castle walls are failing, crumbling, and the wooden structures inside the walls are on fire or already burned. The entire community is ripe for overthrow and domination by an invading force that seems to get stronger every day...

Diversity Is The Key To Stability

I have tried to stress that we, as humans, are not individuals in the sense that we normally think of. We are *self-contained mobile ecosystems* with limited but strong connections to the outside world. Our bodies are the vehicles that contain and transport a tremendous internal world of life through the external environment surrounding us. If we as individuals feel stress, it is likely the microbiome feels stress; if the microbiome is stressed, it is almost certain that our human bodies are affected.

For a microbiome, *stress* is anything that reduces the diversity of the ecosystem. We know from studies in ecology that species diversity in communities is the source of strength for those communities. The loss of species results in several negative consequences for the community. The functions that those species offer to the community are reduced or lost. Think of having a computer keyboard where one of the keys has stopped functioning and how that affects spelling, grammar, and meaning in everything you might try to write. ==The more keys that are missing, the less sense the writing will make.==

A reduction of diversity results in reduced resistance to change. That is, in a highly diverse and inter-connected system, it is difficult to change the system by removing a single piece because all of the other connections can bear the change in stress. But if enough of the system's components are removed or cease to function, the ability of the system to withstand additional stress is lost. (Think about playing Jenga.) Metaphorically speaking, after many subtractions, the loss of one more piece becomes the straw that breaks the camel's back.

Even in highly diverse and inter-connected systems, a great stress can sometimes occur and push the system in a new direction. However, diversity also lends a great degree of resilience to change, and the system can often return to its original state. You've undoubtedly seen a slow-motion video of a ball being struck so hard that the shape of the ball is flattened on one side, but once the ball moves away from the striking force, it regains its original shape. The ball is resilient. It recovers its shape when the stress is removed, just as diverse ecosystems can absorb an environmental stress and recover.

The ability to absorb stress and continue without a loss of function is a form of *plasticity*. It is one of the hallmarks of human physiology: this springy, plastic, resilient characteristic of humans that allows us to live in many harsh environments, eat a tremendous variety of foods, and withstand a barrage of diseases.

While it's true that before about 100 years ago, we were often at the mercy of the environment, and just making it through childhood was one of the great survival filters we faced, the fact is that humans have survived thousands of years of the stresses associated with life in large communities. Today, we have the advantages of advanced technology to protect us from the ravages of the environment, but these "advantages" may also be working against us.

I hope it is now obvious that technology changes the context of our lives as BIGs. It also changes the context of our microbiome, our BUGs, but they are able to adjust almost immediately. However, in the past 75 years, technology has allowed us to dramatically change our context in important ways, and those changes have become constants in our world. They do not allow for the microbiome to "bounce back."

We have reached a point where these major changes to the system are reinforcing other changes and we are witnessing a cascading effect on our health. It's time we recognized that stress after stress after stress to the system might ultimately cause the failure of the system.

I am not saying that modern medicine is bad. You and I are alive because of it. However, the obvious positive effects of such technology often mask subtle negative effects that go unnoticed. The accumulation of these smaller, subtle effects is emerging to reveal real problems, but we are essentially blind to the actual cause-and-effect process because the problems are the result of numerous small changes.

For example, vaccines were first introduced to the public on a large scale after 1900, and by 1930 a number of serious viral and bacterial childhood killers were under control, including diphtheria, typhoid, whooping cough, scarlet fever, and tetanus. The vaccine system is one that introduces some part of the pathogen into the body's system, and the immune system responds. The immune system produces an antigenic response that recognizes the pathogen as foreign and dangerous. That is, we make antibodies against the pathogen, and from that point on, the system is alerted to any future appearances of the pathogenic proteins.

In a healthy body, *the vaccine has educated the immune system* concerning a particular pathogen and thereby prevents that pathogen from overcoming the immune system in the future.

In contrast, antibiotics (introduced in 1945, beginning with penicillin) were also intended to defeat bacterial pathogens but by using a different process. A strong immune system will hunt down and destroy pathogens under normal conditions, but in a weakened system, the body's immune defenses are unable to control the growth of the pathogen, and the result is disease. *Antibiotics provide the missing service* and are essentially an introduced defense system.

However, it is important to recognize the fundamental nature of this interaction. Taking a broad-spectrum antibiotic is akin to hiring a defense contractor who shows up for work only after the walls of the fortress have been breached and many of the houses are already on fire. In addition, the defense contractor shoots indiscriminately at anything resembling the enemy in the belief that collateral damage is not important as long as the enemy is killed. When used appropriately, antibiotics are applied only after the disease has taken hold, and they are tremendously effective at controlling and stopping active bacterial infections, and this saves lives, but it also may come at a cost.

The important difference between vaccines and antibiotics is this: *vaccines strengthen our immune system and antibiotics temporarily replace it*. By using antibiotics, we supplant the multiple natural abilities of the biological system with the single ability of a technological system. It works, but only in the sense that a dangerous pathogen has been stopped. It does not work in the sense that the immune system is strengthened by the experience. Instead, the immune system has been bypassed and perhaps even damaged.

If we accept the recent and compelling research that the microbiome plays an integral role in educating and informing our immune system, and we understand that broad-spectrum antibiotics indiscriminately wipe out any bacteria that have basic similarities to the target pathogen, then the frequent use of antibiotics is weakening our innate ability to defend ourselves from disease.

This happens because by greatly reducing the diversity of the bacteria in our microbiome, we reduce our resistance and resilience, we reduce our immune system's ability to learn and respond, and we reduce our communication with the source of our plasticity, the microbiome. And I say "we" because we as individuals are not separate from the vast bacterial community within us. *"We" are one and the same, and what happens to them also happens to us.*

The actions of antibiotics on our microbiome are indisputable. Martin Blaser[67] has written an eloquent denunciation of antibiotic overuse and misuse and the possible connections with the emergence of certain "modern diseases," such as acid reflux and esophageal cancer. In another review, Pajau Vangay and colleagues [68] summarized the growing evidence for links between disruptions to the microbiome and childhood obesity, autoimmune diseases, allergies, and susceptibility to infectious diseases.

Of particular importance is the evidence that if antibiotic use, and the resulting impairment of the microbiome, occurs during critical developmental stages in infants, the consequences can be permanent. If there was a suspicion that the emergence of modern diseases is directly related to the loss of microbes and microbial diversity in the human microbiome, I think it's safe to say that it is no longer a suspicion as we know it to be true, although we don't know many details of the process.

---

[67] Martin J. Blaser. 2014. *Missing Microbes* (Picador Press). Also M. J. Blaser. 2016. Antibiotic use and its consequences for the normal microbiome. *Science* 352:544-545.

[68] P. Vangay, T. Ward, J.S. Gerber and D. Knights. 2015. Antibiotics, pediatric dysbiosis, and disease. *Cell Host & Microbe* 17:553-564.

Since 1945, antibiotics have become an ingrained part of our lives from birth to death. In 2016, 270 million daily doses were prescribed in the US. Many individuals are taking a course of antibiotics more than once a year. As a species, we had a long and negative history with communicable bacterial diseases, and we adopted antibiotics just as quickly as, well, humanly possible. *We now fear NOT taking antibiotics* when we are faced with an infection or even the possibility of an infection. And the known damage to our system that antibiotics can have is considered a reasonable risk compared to the risk of not taking them.

Antibiotics do one thing and do it well: they kill bacteria. After the slow replacement of the Miasma Theory with the Germ Theory of disease from the mid-1800s to the early 1900s, the deployment of antibiotics in 1945 was probably the single most important event in modern medical history. Unfortunately, we prefer to use broad-spectrum antibiotics because we aren't always sure who the villainous bacterium might be, so we shoot with a shotgun rather than a sniper rifle. Yes, there may be collateral damage, but we know we hit the intended target.

Unfortunately, we are learning, rather slowly and painfully, that the long-term effects of such an approach are, in fact, bad. The effects of the use of broad-spectrum antibiotics can range from zero measurable long-term effects to (potentially) catastrophic influences on health in infants, children, adults, and the elderly by affecting digestion, neural development, and the immune system. But even when it appears there have been zero carryover effects of antibiotic overuse or misuse, we can't ever be sure because those effects may take years to manifest or, more importantly, they may react with other factors in the environment in unpredictable ways.

As I said, this is not to say antibiotics are evil. Quite the contrary! Like vaccines, antibiotics are the reason almost all of us are alive today. At issue is our dependency on a one-size-fits-all battering ram approach for dealing with infections, most of which are not lethal or disabling even when left untreated.

At issue is our love affair with a technology that is applied prophylactically when someone is feeling ill, *just in case,* to prevent the patient from developing a secondary bacterial infection.[69]

---

[69] For example, I recently had minor oral surgery and the periodontist prescribed a broad-spectrum *systemic* antibiotic to prevent an infection *at the site* of the surgery which was between my two front teeth. It is my hope that such prophylactic

And now, we are finding an additional issue in the fact that we have a built-in defense system, the microbiome, that should be working on our behalf to support our health prevent infections, and strengthen our immune systems. *The antibiotics we so casually take may damage the ability of that system to function properly.* Thus, while the use of antibiotics for serious infections can be lifesaving, the routine use of antibiotics should always be tempered by a consideration of the lasting effects it might have on the microbiome and the other systems the microbiome influences.

---

prescriptions will be strongly discouraged by all medical associations within a few years. A second hope would be for the development of more specific antibiotics that can be applied directly to the site of infection.

Chapter 23

Our Chemical Romance

In addition to the concerns over antibiotics and food quality, our modern chemical world must take some heat for the health problems we are having. Simultaneously with the introduction of antibiotics as a public health initiative and the push to genetically "improve" crops for faster growth and higher production, we also introduced an explosion of synthetic chemicals into our environment at every level, from the household to the farm. Thousands of pesticides have been developed in the past 75 years and, in our enthusiasm for the new postwar technological revolution, we just as readily doused ourselves with DDT as we did the fields around us.

Today, the love affair continues: when we leave the house, we spray ourselves, and particularly on our children, with any number of chemicals that we have been told will protect us from the environment. We load up with mosquito sprays, sunscreens, skin lotions, hair sprays, antibacterial lotions, lip glosses, and loads of daily doses of medicines, vitamins, herbals, and tonics. Our clothes, cars, carpets, furniture, and computers are laden with chemicals that emit chemical byproducts. Every object we buy is encased by a variety of plastics, at least half of which are known to produce toxins as they slowly age and break down chemically.

None of these compounds that we are literally inundated with, both awake and asleep, were present before 1950.

Although we can point at antibiotics and some other factors that lead to disease in humans, our clear understanding is hindered because we have not come to grips with the fact that we are not truly individuals in the biological sense. Our individual bodies contain highly complex ecosystems that interact with the host system in uncountable ways. When we argue about the causes of modern diseases, whether in children or adults, we continue to think as we always have. That is, we ask, "What is the single factor responsible for this problem?"

We naively believe that if we can identify that factor, we can eliminate it and cure the problem. Perhaps the pharmaceutical companies can cure us or protect us from the cause. And so, we have been asking simple questions regarding rather complex problems. Are antibiotics to blame? Is our food to blame? Is a chemical to blame?

For all of these questions, the answer is yes, but the problem is that we don't know to what degree. It is not a simple cause-and-effect relationship. The number of variables and the direct and indirect interactions between those variables is staggering. How many variables do we not know about? And of those variables, *time* is the one that science and medicine will never adequately deal with because *time implies a changing context*. Some things may affect us more as an infant than as an adult. It may take years to see the effects of the interactions. Some genotypes among us may react faster than others or not at all. Do some people have "good genes" while others have "bad genes"? Or is it the health of the microbiome and the lack of a million or so bacterial genes?

And so, we find ourselves confused. We are too simple to understand the complexity of ourselves. We are overwhelmed by choices. We aren't sure about believing the health industry when it says a simple pill will cure the problem (if it doesn't also kill you). And we are told to reduce stress and get more sleep because stress exacerbates the problems. That's just great.

However, perhaps the answer is easier than that.

From individual to an ecosystem to the environment

Part of the problem, a big part, is that our thinking about the world is not keeping up with the information we have gathered about the world. Our environmental context has changed, but our viewpoint has not. For example, when rural families move to the city, the parents were born and raised in the country, and their children were born in the country and raised in the city, but the grandchildren are born and raised in the city and think and act like city dwellers. Each extended family possesses a variety of viewpoints about the world and how it works, but each generation is referring to a different set of conditions. It often takes a new generation to truly understand the new environmental context.

We are currently learning a mountain of new information about who we are as biological entities, and we are not able to keep up with it. The information is coming so fast, the breakthroughs of 20 years ago are being re-interpreted in entirely new ways, and we are unable to mentally organize our understanding. As a starting point, we must think about ourselves as biological entities in a different way, and then we can try to see the path forward with that as our new context.

We behave as individuals in every way in our daily lives and this has worked fine for millennia. But the consequences of living in a culture that treats each of us *as if we were no more than an individual* may be a disastrous combination with the other technological changes we have made. In a very real way, the sound you are hearing, the call to arms regarding the state of our environment and the growing number of ugly new diseases in our world, is a call to save ourselves as a species.

Our broader environmental focus is typically on the effects of humans on the ecosystems around us, but it's time to think much more about the effect of our surrounding environment on our health as humans. If we focus on correcting what the environment is doing to our internal ecosystem, we will have taken a huge step toward correcting what we have done to the environment that created this crisis.

At no point in history have our actions literally threatened the entire species, perhaps with the exception of the proliferation of nuclear weapons. But I want to make a point about this: the flood of negative effects we are seeing in our health is related to the microbiome, which is related to everything going on in the external environment in general, both at the microscopic level and at the macroscopic level.

While it has now become necessary for us to focus on the internal microbiome, we cannot ignore the incredible importance of the external microbiome to our internal health. The problem is not specifically the devastation being wrought on the internal microbiome; the problem includes the multiple paths we have taken that have altered our external environment that have brought us to this point.

If I could boil it down to a single word, that word is *simplification*. When humans interact with the world, we simplify it. We reduce natural diversity by eliminating species and environmental complexity. We do this because we redirect the flow of energy in the ecosystem as a way to produce more resources for us.[70] In our less sophisticated days, we were much less able to simplify our surroundings.

Historically, the human population was usually too small to dramatically simplify the world around us, although we certainly tried mightily to do so. History is replete with civilizations that completely transformed their environments, particularly around large cities, but history is also a retelling of how such a transformation often led to the fall of those civilizations.[71]

However, we turned a corner some 250 years ago. The Industrial Revolution, John Deere's invention of the steel the moldboard plow, steam engines, the internal combustion engine, factory-style production systems, and other associated developments accelerated and expanded the intensity of the impacts we could have on our environments. The results weren't just rapidly expanding urban areas, but also the amazingly rapid conversion of diverse wild spaces to simplified cultivated spaces.

Cultivation and agriculture are processes that eliminate the huge diversity of plants and animals in a particular location and replace it with a single species of plant. In agriculture, there is zero interest in any animal presence unless those animals are livestock or pollinators, such as bees. The change in diversity is so profound that the physical conditions of the farmed area are changed. Shade-loving plants die and weeds are favored. Rainfall and sunlight hit the soil directly. The structure of the soil is destroyed by tilling and by the negative effects of sunlight, heat, and dry air on fungi, bacteria, and the many tiny animals. Wind and water erosion strip away the topsoil. Birds, butterflies, spiders, and ladybugs are gone. Literally nothing about the modern farm resembles a natural ecosystem.

While we may think of this as the cost of growing food, our poor understanding of what "healthy" means begins here. What was a healthy ecosystem is now supremely unhealthy. *We grow our food in an ecosystem that we made unhealthy for all other organisms, but we consider it healthy for us.* We modify our crops to reduce genetic variation (an unhealthy thing) and to ramp up the speed of production

---

[70] Carl N. McDaniel and David N. Borton. 2002. Increased human energy use causes biological loss and undermines prospects for sustainability. *BioScience* 52:929-936.

[71] Jared Diamond. 2005. *Collapse: How Societies Choose to Fail or Succeed.* Viking Press.

and at tremendously higher levels of productivity (an unhealthy thing). We don't see the contradictions.

Technology assists us in tweaking and re-tweaking every aspect of food production as we race toward greater and greater production and efficiency with no real acknowledgment of changes in quality as long as the result is changes in quantity. And now we are so far into this way of living, we cannot see the damage we have wrought, we cannot see alternatives, and still we cry out daily for more technology to solve our new problems. Simplification is a problem technology cannot solve. *Simplification is the result of applying technology to complex systems.*

We have taken a similar approach toward the way we feed our bodies. We are told that a normal diet is 1500-2000 calories. The government provides guidelines for what sorts of foods should make up the portions, but with no understanding of how food affects the microbiome or our immune system or how individuals differ from each other. We live in increasing isolation from the environment; all of our food is delivered from an unknown place to our grocery stores. We aren't told that winter produce is from Chile and spring produce is from Mexico or that a rapidly increasing proportion of produce comes from factory-style growing conditions such as greenhouses and hothouses.

We want to believe that food is food in terms of quality and its effects on our bodies and our internal ecosystem. We want to believe that preservatives in our food are protecting us from things that will make us sick. And the list goes on and on, whether we are talking about food, drugs, chemicals, and even the clothes we put on our bodies.

The fact is, our world has changed dramatically, especially in the 75 years since WWII, and we neither know how to judge quality anymore nor who to believe about claims of quality. In fact, those who can remember life before this incredible modernization are at the end of their lives, and the memories of that world will be lost to later generations that never experienced it. Technology has so completely swamped our culture that we have lost our ability to interact with the world in a more natural way. And so, we feel lost and don't even know what to eat or how to protect ourselves from the artificial simplicity that now defines the modern world.

This is where the answers might get easier.

We don't have to look outward for diversity and complexity in a highly simplified world. Each of us possesses it inherently, and it can respond and re-emerge literally overnight. A recent film provides an example of the strength of our internal ecosystem and how those species will work day and night to maintain the health of their own ecosystem.

In the documentary film "*Fat, Sick, and Nearly Dead*" (2010), Joe Cross changes his life and then the lives of others, using an entirely plant-based juice diet. The primary focus of the diet is to lose weight and regain control over health, and this works because of the immense increase in food quality and plant-based nutrients for those people on the juice diet.

However, what almost certainly happened with the switch from the highly processed Western Diet to a plant-based diet consisting entirely of fresh produce was the massive increase of minerals and vitamins for the body and food diversity to the starved microbiomes in the dieters. While the juice diet does not include most of the indigestible plant material, it does include a significant amount of fiber and plant chemicals.

That massive shift from nearly 0% to 100% prebiotic content was guaranteed to shift the composition and complexity of the dieters' microbiomes. Among other changes in health status was the disappearance of some auto-immune problems and allergies, which had nothing to do with the diet *per se*. These changes were almost certainly the consequence of consuming higher quality nutrients that supported a healthier microbiome.

What this movie exemplifies is that life in this simplified, technological, polluted world can be healthier, even for a 430-pound truck driver, with a relatively simple change to a diet that more closely resembles the diet of our country-living grandparents and great-grandparents. That is a shift toward a fresher, plant-based, higher-quality diet. OK, but before we get to that, let me take a slightly different tack because merely eating fresh produce is not the entire story here.

Chapter 24

Repairing The Damage And Restoring Health

Prior to 1900, almost all of the corn eaten in the US was processed using the Native American alkali or lime method (called *nixtamalization*). Shortly after 1900, corn processing changed to the *degermination method* in which the germ (corn embryo) was removed prior to milling the grain. The main purpose for the change was that the oils in the germ tended to degrade quickly and the shelf life of the ground corn was short. The rancid oils gave the corn a bad smell. (To experience the smell of rancid corn oil, open an old bag of corn chips and breathe deeply.). Unfortunately, the germ also contains all of the beneficial oils and nutrients other than starch.

Almost immediately, an interesting disease broke out (mostly) in the southern United States among the poorest people in the region: pellagra.[72] This disease is identified by the 3 D's: Dermatitis, Diarrhea, and Delirium, which are followed by a fourth D: Death. Victims with advanced cases of pellagra were often committed to insane asylums as a result of the delirium, and the Southern asylums quickly became overcrowded with large numbers of patients.

With a death rate of about 40%, as many as 10,000 people were dying each year by 1915, and as many as 100,000 deaths from 3 million cases occurred over the course of about 30 years. Officials at every level looked high and low for the culprit, which they felt had to be a pathogen, but no bacterial or viral agent could be associated with

---

[72] For a detailed summary of the pellagra epidemic, see Alfred Jay Bollet. 1992. Politics and Pellagra: The epidemic of pellagra in the U.S. in the early twentieth century. *Yale Journal of Biology and Medicine* 65:211-221.

the disease. In no small way, the insistence of politicians and administrators on looking only for an infectious source was the largest obstacle to solving the problem.

The Southern states were still recovering from the disastrous cultural and economic effects of the Civil War, and politicians were very sensitive to any implication that the South was anything but modern and equal to states in the North. Thus, any suggestion that pellagra could be a result of malnutrition in regions that were actually net producers of food was considered an insult and was summarily dismissed as an underlying cause of the problem.

However, the eventual discovery and later acceptance of the source of the problem was the basic diet of poor Southerners: the 3M diet, which was meat, molasses, and meal. The typical affordable diet among the poor was corn meal (starch) and cane syrup (sugar) supplemented by fatty pork when it was available. Ultimately, the cause of pellagra was found to be a near absence of niacin (Vitamin B_3), and this was a result of the shift to the degermination method of processing corn, which eliminated the most common natural source of niacin (and tryptophan) in the 3M diet.

The pellagra epidemic is a good example of a subtle dietary change that had profound effects on public health.[73] The change was no more than a modernization of the way we handled one common food component (corn) in our diet. Of course, as soon as the source of the problem was recognized, we stopped processing corn in that manner, and the problem with pellagra disappeared. No, I'm just kidding. We didn't change anything. We still process most corn in that manner, but we make sure to add vitamins back into the meal. In fact, the reason so many of our grain-based foods are labeled as "enriched," such as almost everything containing wheat flour, is precisely because of this legacy of pellagra and the intentional removal of important nutrients for more efficient processing and longer shelf life.

This, in fact, may be the source of our current health problems more than any other cause: the food industry is convinced (and fervently wishes to convince us) that food supplemented with nutrients is the same as the real deal. Michael Pollan has written

---

[73] Another example is the beriberi outbreaks in Japan in the late 1800s. Thiamine (Vitamin B_1) deficiency resulted from a diet high in polished white rice because the natural vitamins in the rice had been removed in the polishing process. Like the pellagra epidemic, the victims had a diet high in calories, but low in nutrients.

extensively on this problem of looking at "food" as a combination of nutrients.[74]

All of us are guilty of thinking that taking a supplement (for example, a daily vitamin) is more or less equivalent to balancing an otherwise unbalanced diet. We accept the constant barrage of advice from the food, drug, and supplement industries who suggest that merely adding a missing component is the same as eating actual food and that taking a medicine that replaces a function is the same as having the natural function. And now we're adding the microbiome as just another layer on top of the artificial edifice we call our modern diet.

The Big Picture Is The Big Problem

As we try to get a handle on food and the microbiome and what that means for our health, we find there is an additional twist that we must recognize and respect. We are trying to juggle the multiple variables involved, *but they all seem to be changing at the same time*; the sand is shifting under our feet. We have modified every aspect of our social, cultural, and natural environment, but we are drifting further and further away from what our bodies understand naturally. While we may feel that making such adjustments is easy, our physiological and microbiome selves may not be nearly as amenable to some of these changes.

In some way or another, most of the changes to our environment have been changes in chemistry. The microbiome is a chemical world; the bacteria in the microbiome live in and understand a chemical world. We, as humans, do not. We try hard to recognize which chemicals are directly harmful to our physiology, but we do not understand and will not understand, until it is way too late, just how chemicals affect us in indirect ways.

By the time we identify a complex health syndrome, we are typically too far into the weeds to be able to tease apart the many different factors that have contributed to the disease. It takes years to recognize the subtle environmental changes that lead to health complications, and by the time we do, if we do, we have made many additional changes to the environment. The good news is that the microbiome can probably tell us within hours to weeks what chemical changes are negative. We have to listen, though. And even more than

---

[74] Michael Pollan. 2008. *In Defense of Food*. Penguin Press

that, we have to let the microbiome tell us what chemical changes are positive, and this is a focus we have neglected until today.

The fad diets, including the FDA/USDA guidelines, are all focused on food with the goal of avoiding "the bad stuff" and emphasizing "the good stuff." Quite often, we think of a "good" diet as one that doesn't have overtly "bad" things in it *rather than approaching the issue in exactly the opposite way*. The definition of good and bad has been notoriously difficult to determine. Pinpointing obviously "bad" foods is like labeling a particular bacterium as "bad": that is, it's entirely contextual.

Until recently, the American Medical Association had worked assiduously (and struggled mightily) to create and modify recommendations regarding the best practices for avoiding and reducing a serious health problem in America. Finally, the AMA threw in the towel and now just says, "we have no recommendation." The bad guy? Dietary cholesterol.

After decades of chasing this hoodlum to collect evidence of wrongdoing, the medical and science detectives have failed to get a conviction. Why? Because cholesterol is a natural and absolutely necessary component of our system. Our bodies make cholesterol and, if we don't eat enough, our bodies compensate by making more. There are no effective ways to modify the diet to consistently and predictably lower blood cholesterol and yet we know that high blood cholesterol is linked to cardiovascular disease. So, is there no solution? Are we doomed?

The AMA says simply: exercise more. Why? *Because exercise changes the context.* Exercise changes the internal physiological environment in a hundred different direct and indirect ways. And people who exercise routinely also change their lifestyle, and that means what they eat, how much, and when. And the quality of the food goes up when we are paying attention to how food makes us feel and when we are taking responsibility for our health. Similarly, when we are conscious of our health, it is easier to follow the basic admonition: "excess is bad, moderation is good."

The failure of the AMA to design written-in-stone recommendations for managing blood cholesterol should be seen as a *positive outcome*. It reflects a shift (albeit minor) in the medical world from attempting to explain our health as a function of single variables. Of course, there are single variables that greatly affect our health, such as pathogens like the Ebola virus and Bubonic Plague bacteria. But diseases that take years to manifest (such as cardiovascular diseases) and that only some people get are likely the result of a great many environmental factors. The recommendation to *change your lifestyle* is a recommendation to *change your context,* and that means to change not one but a great many variables in a positive way. While the many people who were hoping for a silver bullet cure for high cholesterol may not think so, I see the AMA recommendation as a success story.

Humans are complex. We are more complex than pure carnivores and pure herbivores. We are omnivores; we live in and experience a variable and unpredictable dietary environment. Michael Pollan has described this "dilemma" faced by omnivores in terms of choosing food as a source of confusion for our society. However, I suggest that omnivory *allows us* to live in that variable and unpredictable dietary environment, but it *requires us* to maintain a tremendously flexible digestive capacity. We can eat all manner of foods that are not explicitly toxic, but that resiliency and flexibility demands a rapid response system and one is capable of adjusting to novelty.

So, for humans, are there good and bad foods? We have been told daily (and for decades) that there are definitely bad foods. Yes, fats are bad! OK, but shouldn't cultures that eat oily meats as a major part of their diet have died out? Well then, dairy fats! OK, but then cheese should have brought down the French. Ummm, coconut oil? Hmmm, then all Pacific islands should be uninhabited. How about carbs from grains? Then all Middle Easterners are doomed.

Every culture has a food emphasis that has at one time or another been considered "bad," but those cultures live on healthily. The Western world is obsessed with food choices because we are eliminating basic foods, historical choices, and nutritional quality. More to the point, we are being told that the food substitutes are equal to the real thing, AND we are being sold foods that appear to be the real thing but aren't.

The bottom line is that naturally occurring food is food. Food that we have been exposed to for hundreds and thousands of years is food. "Food" that has emerged in the past 70-100 years might not be food. And we are confused about the differences. There are two items that we must deal with regarding food. Both are crucial to living a healthy life in the modern world. First, we have to understand *who we are* when it comes to food. Second, we have to be able *to recognize food.*

Chapter 25

Thinking Like An Ecosystem

We have to think differently. It's time to think not like 8 billion human individuals but as a species that understands who we are and how we got to where we are. The human world has changed in the past 10,000 years for one simple reason: we have advanced our technological prowess to the point that we let technology and science make decisions for us. We especially love science and technology when we get what we desire.

However, it's important to note that there exists a basic misunderstanding of the difference between science and technology. The confusion is really the difference between basic science and applied science. Basic science is a process for discovery and understanding, and it is impersonal in the sense that scientific decisions are based on facts rather than desire.

For example, when evolutionary biologists announced in the 1950s that insect resistance to pesticides and bacterial resistance to penicillin were clear demonstrations of the Principle of Natural Selection, we did not listen because that was not the voice we wanted to hear.

Simultaneously, the applied science world (technology) was proclaiming that the early problems with pest control were expected symptoms of the trial-and-error process of basic science and that new information would result in improved technological solutions.

The voice of applied science was the voice we wanted to hear. This voice promised the kind of world we thought we wanted to live in. This world is one where humans are in charge of everything, Nature must submit to our desires, and Science is the tool for achieving those desires.

And so, our burgeoning population (one that grew from 1.6 billion in 1900 to 2.5 billion in 1945 to nearly 8 billion today) has continued to think as it has always thought. We worry about people as individuals, we worry about food as something that keeps our bodies alive, and we readily accept whatever technology can offer to assist us. And we are missing a big point.

Humans are not individuals. Not in a biological sense. This failure to understand who we are as organisms is at the root of the problems we face as a species in the 21st Century.

Humans are somewhat self-contained mobile ecosystems containing many trillions of partners within our microbiomes. The terrestrial macro-ecosystems surrounding us create the context through which we move. Like all animals, we are "somewhat self-contained" in that each of us is an independently moving ecosystem, but also one that actively makes exchanges with the external ecosystem, albeit through highly filtered exchanges. Under stable conditions, we don't really need inputs from the external world (other than food). If our food environment never changed, we could probably exist quite well without added inputs from the outside.

Unfortunately, our world is not stable. We experience constant flux in terms of the kinds of food we eat, the pathogens we are exposed to, and the chemicals in our environment that affect our bodies and our internal ecosystems. And while our internal ecosystems are resistant and resilient, our modern technological world now wields large hammers that are capable of completely restructuring the microbiome almost instantaneously.

Antibiotics are just such a hammer. One by one, each antibiotic eventually fails through bacterial resistance, but we make bigger and better hammers to satisfy our (still) naïve impulse to define the rules of life. In terms of medicine, the release of penicillin in 1945 was the biggest hammer blow to disease in history. It hit the bacteria living in the human body hard, and almost nothing stood in its path.

The unpleasant side effects on humans could also be quite fierce: nausea, vomiting, diarrhea, abdominal pain, rashes and itching, thrush, swollen tongue, headache, and occasionally anaphylaxis, seizures, and anemia. For a medicine that kills a wide range of presumably unnecessary bacteria, that's quite a list of *negative* responses for a human suffering from the effects of only one of those bacteria. Perhaps we should have wondered more about that.

Doctors like to use antibiotic hammers because, quite often, the exact pathogen causing a health problem is not known, so "kill all to get one" is considered a reasonable approach. After all, they're just bacteria. And it usually works. Pharmaceutical companies also like big hammers because they want to sell something that can be used in a variety of situations. The unfortunate reality of the pharmaceutical world is that the development of specific antibiotics is just as expensive as that of broad-spectrum antibiotics. However, the narrow spectrum drug will sell fewer units, and therefore each unit must be more expensive for the consumer.

And so, doctors often prescribe broad-spectrum antibiotics for general malaise. That is, if a patient is feeling poorly and there isn't an obvious connection to a pathogen, a doctor's approach is that a broad-spectrum antibiotic will cover a lot of territory, it won't do any particular harm, the patient will feel better about being treated, and the patient almost always recovers (anyway) in a few days.

In fact, most pediatricians know that 90% of the children being brought in as "sick" will recover within a few days to a week whether or not the doctor prescribes anything. This is because most childhood illnesses are viral, and kids usually have great immune systems. Because the child and especially the parent would like to have a prescription, it would make more sense for doctors to default to a placebo rather than to antibiotics, which are prescribed inappropriately about 36% of the time (CDC, 2016 data).

The fact that patients almost always recover is a testament to the strength and resilience of the immune system and, therefore, to the microbiome. However, the current medical system is dominated by worries of malpractice suits; if the doctor failed to prescribe an antibiotic and the patient contracted an unrelated secondary infection, the legal consequences for the doctor would be catastrophic. Better to prescribe the antibiotic; no harm done.

But what happens when the antibiotic fails or makes matters worse? When an antibiotic fails to eliminate a bacterial problem, the typical approach is to prescribe a different broad-spectrum antibiotic and to keep doing so until the patient shows signs of improvement. In cases of a stubborn illness, even intravenous antibiotics may be given. While this approach may ultimately and apparently eliminate the stubborn pathogen, the serial application of strong antibiotics can be disastrous for the microbiome and can lead to life-threatening conditions.

For example, consider *Clostridioides difficile* or *C. diff*. Chronic and untreatable *C. diff* infections[75] and the increasingly favored cure for that infection may be the most talked-about example of the relationship between the microbiome and intestinal disorders and perhaps the best example of a reason for changing some current medical practices.

The difficult thing to understand is how and why *C. diff* becomes such a problem. It is one disease that is clearly linked to serial antibiotic use and to particular antibiotics.[76] We know that a series of different antibiotics can (apparently) facilitate the infection and can also make an existing infection worse. Both outcomes are clearly linked to the major disruption of the gut microbiome by the antibiotics. We know that stopping antibiotic treatment does not make the problem go away, which means the microbiome has been so disturbed that it cannot right itself. The standard treatment is more antibiotics, but even those antibiotics that are known to be effective against *C. diff* fail a significant percentage of the time.

We also know that *C. diff* did not become a problem merely because it was introduced to the system and just took over. No, *C. diff* is a relatively common resident in the large intestine, just like the common cold virus in our noses and *Streptococcus* bacteria in our throats. Something facilitated the change in ecosystem balance; something weakened the system and allowed *C. diff* to become dominant and entrenched. *C. diff* is an opportunistic pathogen that lies in wait until the conditions are favorable for a coup, an overthrow of the system, but the system must be greatly weakened first. This happens when the microbiome is simplified and isolated from the outside world. Reversing the dominance of *C. diff* is not easy. Unfortunately, a large input of beneficial and diverse bacteria from the food we eat (i.e., probiotics) is an unlikely occurrence because of the strong filters as bacteria pass through the upper digestive system.

Fortunately, there is another way for a massive input of bacteria to arrive in the lower digestive tract. We now know that the most effective way of treating *C. diff* is a fecal transplant, that is, seeding a

---

[75] The number of *C. diff* infections is rising, but estimates vary by year and source. The CDC estimated *C. diff* infections at nearly 500,000 in 2015 with 100,000 in nursing homes. The Mayo Clinic estimates 200,000 per year in nursing homes and another 170,000 outside of health care facilities. Both sources agree the numbers are rising.

[76] C.G. Buffie and E.G. Pamer. 2013. Microbiota-mediated colonization resistance against intestinal pathogens. *Nature Reviews Immunology* 13:790-801.

healthy microbiome into the damaged system. While the mere suggestion of a fecal transplant will raise a few eyebrows, a better than 90% success rate – much higher than the antibiotic success rate – should allay those concerns. When a strong herbicide is applied to a pasture and kills all of the plants there, the only way to re-establish the plants is from seed. Likewise, when the microbial community in a colon has been so devastated by a series of antibiotics that even the appendix can't restart the system, a large infusion of bacteria from a healthy colon is the best (and sometimes only) answer.

C. diff is just one example of the importance of having a diverse ecosystem in our colon and also an example of the resilience of the system and the human body. Even after months of disease and damage from *C. diff*, the system can be restored and it can happen within hours to a few days. Unfortunately, *C. diff* is also just one of many examples of the damage we are causing to the microbiome when we consider antibiotics to be the best and sometimes the only tool in the toolbox.

And again, when we see *C. diff* in a patient, we have little to no understanding of the influence of age, developmental stage, personal history, genetics, and diet on the severity of the disease. What we can see is this: applying a series of drugs (i.e., technology) that are hugely destructive to bacteria seems to have facilitated an apparently incurable disease, but one that can be cured almost instantaneously by reinstating the diverse bacterial community from a healthy person's colon. What do we learn from a lesson that essentially is this: the cure for a bacterial problem is more bacteria?

If it is true that we are each highly diverse, dynamic, contextual, independent ecosystems and the health of the host absolutely depends on the care of that ecosystem, then how should we live as humans? How do we maintain our health in a world that is changing faster than we even know? Perhaps more importantly, what do we eat for lunch?

If you watch TV, you already know this is a multi-billion-dollar question, and the food and drug companies are earnestly trying to convince you they know the answers. (Hint: they don't.) They are operating on only the tiniest of clues. The scientists actively researching the microbiome and human health don't have a handle on it. The surface has just been scratched, the first layers of the onion have been peeled back, and we're still in the "counting on our fingers" stage of documenting the diversity and some of the more obvious interactions.

The good news is that the problem for you and me is not as complicated. We don't actually have to understand the microbiome for us to be active caretakers. We know that the microbiome is not an accidental assemblage of bacteria, that it has been there for ages, that it may be crucial to our digestive processes, and that some of the bacteria are providing nutritional and protective services. We know that diversity is good and simplification is bad. We know that the microbiome feeds on plant material and that food diversity supports bacterial diversity. We know that flexibility in the face of change is an asset and that diverse systems are more flexible.

We know many of the basic rules of external ecosystems and we can pretty safely assume that such rules apply to the internal ecosystem. Let's take the rules we know from external ecosystems and apply them to our microbiome.

Chapter 26

Eating Like An Ecosystem

"Let me explain. No, it's too much. Let me sum up."
                                  -Inego Montoya (*The Princess Bride*)

Michael Pollan summarized his advice for eating well in seven words: *Eat food, not too much, mostly plants.*[77] He arrived at that advice without considering the microbiome. But if we have to think about eating in terms of feeding the microbiome, then what? In my opinion, *nothing*. Pollan's advice about feeding the human body is probably the perfect advice for feeding the microbiome too.

In his view, "eating food" means eating food that resembles the original organism, which is to say, is not highly processed and still possesses most of the original qualities in terms of vitamins, minerals, fiber, and so on. In other words, the food should be as natural as possible and not be covered by the fingerprints (read: enhancements) of technology. And Pollan insisted that plants should be the basis of the diet, and those plants should be as fresh and natural as possible.

Let's go back to the tomato. I suggested that the tomato fruit is the expression of the tomato genome and that the garden tomato is the fullest expression of that genetic potential. The garden tomato contains everything that a tomato plant is capable of having because it has been challenged by the garden environment to express all of those attributes it has collected over evolutionary time in response to all manner of environmental stresses. In much the same way, our microbiome has incredible potential hidden in the thousands of species represented by trillions of bacteria possessing an estimated five million genes. What does it take to unlock that potential and to

---
[77] Pollan 2008.

take advantage of the incredible ability of bacteria to produce new mutations rapidly?

The key to microbiome health is the partnership with bacteria and the realization that they are not alien hitchhikers but digestive partners. They *belong* in our colon. We literally invited them in. The colon is an odd organ, but close examination reveals that it is an ideal housing complex for bacteria, and quite possibly, we have a backward opinion of it.

The indigestible parts of the food we eat pass quickly through the small intestine to the colon. The colon is sealed from the oxygenated environment and is ideal for fermentation. The appendix is situated where it can influence the composition of the colon quickly. Food passage is slow and deliberate, and the conditions change from one end to the other, which creates varying habitats for supporting community diversity. *The colon is an ideal bacterial environment.*

Importantly, absorption of nutrients is not the primary function of the colon, which is in stark contrast to the small intestine, where absorption is definitely the primary function. The environment of the colon is not designed for food digestion in the same way that chemical secretion in the small intestine denatures carbs, fats, and proteins. No, the colon is a place where our digestive enzymes don't even serve a purpose.

As humans, we have a limited chemical arsenal when it comes to digesting food material, but our colon is a place where the biochemical arsenal is almost limitless, and the toughest materials and chemical compounds in our food can be degraded. The structure of the colon is ideal for that task, but only if the attacking hordes are bacteria. It has to be bacteria.

The omnivore diet of humans can literally contain any kind of food material, and the plant components will vary on an almost monthly basis if one eats what is naturally available. Hunter and gatherer humans were mobile and moved frequently to follow the seasonal food supply, and pastoralist and agricultural cultures also cultivated and ate a wide variety of plant foods. Spicy, aromatic, and even toxic plants were incorporated into regional cuisines, which added more chemical complexity. Plants are everywhere, which means food is everywhere, but only if it can be digested. How to handle the digestive chores faced by omnivorous humans? It has to be bacteria.

So, we must feed our partners. *We must eat for an ecosystem.* That's the rub: if we think of ourselves as individuals, our approach to eating is simple, but if we think of ourselves as ecosystems, our approach to eating should be very different. The simple approach is to think that for nutrition, we need proteins, fats, and carbs in some kind of proportion, and for health, we avoid the overconsumption of calories. And fiber is indigestible, but it keeps everything moving. Simple, right?

Most of us just worry about the proportions of proteins, fats, and carbs. At different times in recent history, proteins, fats, and carbs have all been considered good or bad, and to the point today that we aren't sure who to listen to. And as we try to decide, we also are told that the quality of the foods we eat has changed. Wheat is now laden with gluten, cows are fed exclusive corn, the flavor is disappearing, chicken has antibiotics, produce is grown under sterile conditions in hothouses, and so on. What to do? What to eat? Eating as an individual used to be easy! Now we're fat and tired and allergic and stressed, and exercise doesn't seem to help. Perhaps it's not so simple anymore.

Or maybe it is. If we eat to feed an ecosystem, we change the focus from feeding ourselves to eating what supports "them." "They" need plants, fiber, and diversity, and not proteins, fats, and carbs. The microbiome needs us to eat food that can make it through the small intestine to their anaerobic home in the colon. This needs to be our new normal everyday diet and it needs to vary constantly in composition.

Our diet should be a flow of food information from the outside world. The food we eat should not be a single favorite plant that favors the dominance of only certain bacteria; it should be a buffet. It should be fruits and vegetables, leaves and roots, seeds and flowers, nuts and berries. It should not be peeled, canned, mechanically processed, or cooked unto death in oil. Flavors should not have to be added except to enhance the natural flavors of the plant, and added flavors should be plant-based. Our plant-based diet should be full of strong flavors. Remember, eating isn't about you personally; eating is about you collectively.

Chapter 27

Food Quality And Why It Matters

Some confusion is to be expected as to what healthy eating means. As easy as "just eat lots of plants" might seem, the agriculture and food industries have been working assiduously against the success of such a simple approach to eating. In some cases, the changes to our crops have been on purpose, and in most cases, it's a result of marketing for nationwide and global sales. Since the 1950s, our modern approach to agriculture has been focused on pesticides, fertilizer, giant fields of a single crop, and breeding for complete genetic and physical uniformity. None of this is in the best interest of food quality and human health.

While it's true that the broader intent was to provide large quantities of inexpensive food to the growing US and global populations, the method for achieving that goal was to simplify the process to the greatest extent possible.[78] With the development of genetic technologies, food science chemistry, and the shift in agribusiness to large food corporations, many of our crop plants and animals are no more than delivery systems for the proteins, fats, and carbs that make up the "simple" diet.

Now our protein is produced in massive feed lots for cattle, pigs, chickens, and fish where genetically uniform animals are more-or-less force-fed an unnatural and uniform diet (of mostly corn products). These animals grow and reach maturity rapidly and are processed even more rapidly in highly efficient factory situations. Carbs and fats in our diet are derived from wheat, corn, and soybeans grown in

---

[78] *Chasing the Red Queen* (Dyer 2014) was a review of the different aspects of this process and the harm it has caused to the environment.

massive acreages of genetic uniformity and then processed so the chemical components can be extracted and used as part of the processed food industry.

Of course, I have an issue with modern agriculture and the industrial way in which we produce "food," but the long-term issues are what that technology does to the food itself (not to mention the environment!). For us to eat a healthy diet, we are faced with grocery stores full of produce that has come increasingly from a commercial food-production system that is essentially industrial and focused on efficiency and marketability and has no particular interest in quality other than appearance.

Indeed, legal challenges to the modern style of food production, specifically of genetic modification of crops, usually fall flat because the food industry can and does argue that there are no "significant" differences between traditional crops and modern crops. This argument is disingenuous at best, but it means that if one were to look at the biochemistry of the food item, one would find that the same chemicals are found in both, and therefore they are not different. A steak from a feedlot cow is not different from a steak from a grass-fed cow. GMO field corn is not chemically different from wild corn.

This is a difficult argument to beat because the definition of healthy vs. unhealthy is poorly considered and poorly understood. We can't beat that argument because we lack the understanding of how the human ecosystem handles and reacts to basic, even subtle, shifts in food quality. Similarly, as humans age, our nutrient requirements change; what we need as children is not the same as when we are fully mature adults. The food industry treats all humans alike, just as the USDA Food Plate (formerly the Food Pyramid and the Food Wheel) treats us all as if we were the same age, and with a hard-to-understand emphasis on carbs (from grains) in our diets.

So, how do we handle the confusion over food choices? It would help to have a better understanding of who we are genetically. First, the historical diet of humans, as recently as 10,000 years ago, had almost no grains in it except perhaps as a seasonal part of the diet. That changed slowly for Asian and Mediterranean cultures with the advent of agriculture and sedentary societies and the year-round presence of grains in the diet. Some ethnicities (for example, African, Australian, Native American, Aleuts, and Peoples of the North) have little to no history with these types of carbs.

Second, dairy products are a part of many but by no means all cultures. Lactose intolerance is an indicator for many ethnicities of a historical absence of milk products. Third, the dentition of humans is clearly adapted for chewing and grinding, not for cutting and tearing, and this indicates to anthropologists that plants have long formed the basis of the human diet. While some cultures may have migrated in the distant past to places where meat provides the majority of their calories, the longer historical evidence supports a plant-based diet that was supplemented by meat. Fourth, our discussion of the structure of the colon and the microbiome it contains is an incredibly clear indicator of the overwhelming importance of plants, not meats, in the diet.

Food for humans starts with plants (excluding carb-rich grains.) Until a few decades ago, those plants were a diverse mixture and regionally grown, each was genetically diverse and grown in relatively small patches on small farms, and all plants were valued for their flavors.[79] They weren't "organically grown" because that label had no meaning; most foods were organically grown, and it wasn't until the advent of artificial fertilizers and pesticides (and antibiotics and hormones for animals) after WWII that food crops weren't "organic." All food was natural and organic and a product of the soil.

Thus, if we are to consider what healthy food is, we have to understand our relationship to the production of food and then what the changes in the production of food in the past 70 years have done to that food. When we choose food in the market, we should think about the plants that make up that food, yes, but also about how those plants have been grown and harvested.

So, to recap:

*Each of us houses a thousand different species of bacteria in our gut and each species has a particular food preference.

*We must therefore provide a range of food for our bacterial health and prosperity.

*We must also eat for ourselves, but our food choices should be informed and deliberate, and this need is only accentuated by the ease with which we can make poor choices in today's world.

---

[79] A great introduction to this topic is *Southern Provisions: The Creation and Revival of a Cuisine* by David S. Shields (University of South Carolina), who has worked for decades to find the original food resources of the south that contained flavors now missing in their modern counterparts. He maintains that true Southern cuisine can only be made with the proper ingredients, such as the rice, beans, and sugars, that have the flavors of old because they are grown from the right cultivars in the right soils and in the right climate.

*We must also remember that we and our microbiome possess tremendous resilience and flexibility. Our microbiome can adjust to changes in the diet on the fly, literally overnight. Short-term negative events are not a problem, but chronic shortages and insults are.

*The human body is equally tough, although probably because the microbiome is there to help us.

And so, depending on our current health status, none of our food is poisonous in small doses no matter how it was produced, how genetically modified it is, how processed it is, or how much high fructose corn syrup it contains. We can take antibiotics and not suffer long-term digestive disorders, but it is likely that our susceptibility may depend on our personal diet patterns (and a number of poorly understood aspects of our personal history). Our physiological resilience means we can endure insults to our system and not lose our normal functions. We have survived thousands of years of dietary uncertainty and pestilence and famine, and our microbiome has been our partner the entire way. And here we are.

But we, as a species (of individual self-contained mobile ecosystems), are under chronic attack and that's a problem because our microbiome is under that same attack. We live in an environment that appears to be reducing our resilience and resistance, one that is weakening our ability to repel invaders, and we are exposed to an ever-increasing toxic external environment that is also losing its resistance and resilience. We must act, and the first step is to understand what food is and use that understanding to maintain our health.

Chapter 28

Getting Your Diet In Order

We have been obsessed with diets for decades, but especially since the 1950s. Year by year, our fad diets have been getting more sophisticated and more "science-based" in terms of the specificity of the recommendations and the reasons behind them. Some diet plans focus on specially prepared (often highly processed) foods and others have shifted towards more natural foods. Some diets provide guidelines for eating and leave the specific decisions to the dieter and other plans are very prescriptive.

None of the fad diets are effective for the majority of the participants and this is most often blamed on difficulties sticking to the diet. This seems strange because it really shouldn't be hard to eat right, to feel full, and to stick to a meal plan, and it shouldn't be hard to maintain a healthy weight that doesn't fluctuate wildly. Yes, our body shape does change as we age, especially as we become less active, but disease should not be a normal expectation of aging.

At this point, we've covered a lot of ground about the microbiome, evolutionary biology, ecology, and ecosystems, but what do a few trillion bacteria in our colon have to do with our diet plan? We are learning that our microbiome doesn't just live in the colon, and its influence extends throughout the body. It communicates with the immune system and the brain, and it supports itself by supporting us.

We will never know all there is to know, but we know enough to be good stewards of the microbiome, which in turn is adapted to support the ecosystem in which it resides. We know enough to make smart dietary decisions, which means we can make smart health decisions.

Our diet should focus first on microbiome support and second on metabolic support.

Microbiome support: As we consider what to eat on a daily basis, we should first consider what the microbiome needs to be balanced, diverse, informed, and that means the majority of our diet should be plants. Not plant-based, mind you, but actual plants. What we want to get from plants can be quite diverse, but our *number one criterion is fiber*, which is to say cellulose. Cellulose is the structural component of plants that we, as humans, cannot digest, and it will move quickly through our upper digestive tract to the colon. Cellulose is the foundation on which the microbiome is built because it is the material that provides the microbiome with an energy source.

Cellulose is by far the most abundant of the huge variety of molecules in plants that support the microbiome. The qualities of cellulose differ from plant to plant. Pure cellulose is a polysaccharide made by linking together glucose (sugar) molecules, but cellulose can contain other related substances like pectin, hemicellulose, and lignin. These components vary in abundance in the cellulose molecule, and that variation is key to the qualities of fiber from different plants. Bacteria tend to be specialists at breaking down particular molecular components of cellulose and therefore, a diverse plant diet can support a greater diversity of bacterial types.

Metabolic support: In addition to cellulose for support of the microbiome, our diet should provide calories to support our metabolic needs. Those calories come as proteins, fats, and carbohydrates – let's call them the PFC portion of our diet – and we all need about 1500-2000 calories per day for our resting metabolism. The more physically active we are, the higher our metabolic rate and the more calories we need to consume.

However, these calories are not useful to the bacteria in the microbiome. Under normal circumstances, the PFC food materials are broken down rapidly, absorbed in the small intestine, and never make it to the colon. So, our obsession with counting calories and PFC grams in our diet should always take a back seat to our primary goal of providing cellulose materials to the microbiome.

What this means is that fad diets that claim certain types of food are "bad" are making the wrong point that our primary concern relating to the diet is calories. The "good" and "bad" foods that are the focus of all fad diets are always PFC foods and never plants. The "bad" foods are highly unlikely to be overtly bad for you (excluding allergens, perhaps), but the emphasis on PFC is itself indicative of a poorly balanced diet *with respect to the source of your health*, which is the microbiome.

Nonetheless, we have to eat PFC foods to support our metabolic energy demands (and because they're delicious), so condemning some of them makes no sense, nor does trying to replace them with nutritional supplements. Supplements are not food, and the supposed need for supplements again masks an imbalance in the makeup of the diet. With few exceptions, every nutritional supplement we take is derived from a plant, and the need for plant-based supplements implies a lack of appropriate plant material in the diet. And so, let's take the villains out of this story and focus instead on the heroes.

To sum up, everyone's obsession with calories in the diet is based on an incorrect view of what in our diet makes us healthy.

*The indigestible portion of our food is always plant materials, and it's the only part that feeds the microbiome. A healthy rule when eating any meal is to feed the microbiome first and feed yourself second.

*The focus on proteins, fats, and carbs is a focus on the calories that provide energy and building blocks for the physical body. These materials provide *nothing* for the microbiome, but are a great source of income for those selling fad diets.

*The need for vitamins and minerals is an indicator of an imbalanced diet that lacks fresh plant materials. Supplements do not replace fresh plants in the diet.

Chapter 29

Real Food Is Slow Medicine

"Virtually all of the major tomato volatiles can be linked to compounds providing health benefits to humans."[80]

There is little scientific evidence to support claims that chemical extracts from plants act as rapid and effective medicines. Herbal supplements do not (and cannot) overtly claim that cancers or allergies or other diseases can be prevented, reduced, or cured. This isn't to say that plants can't or don't have these qualities, but unfortunately our comparison system is one that is oriented around modern chemical medicine. To date, research on plant-based supplements has provided little evidence for substantial changes in metabolic and physiologic processes in comparison to synthetic medicines designed for addressing specific medical issues.

This is true. And it misses the point.

Medicines are short-term technological solutions for acute biological problems. Medicines are designed to replace biological processes whenever the body is unable to overcome a dangerous situation or condition. Medicines rarely boost the natural processes of the body. In fact, those medicines taken for chronic health issues are not intended to correct the medical problem and *are used as permanent substitutes*.

New medicinal compounds are tested for rapid effectiveness, for low toxicity, and for obvious side effects, and the testing period is rarely longer than 2-3 years because the development and testing of new medicines is incredibly expensive. There is an implicit

---

[80] S.A. Goff and H.J. Klee. 2006. Plant volatile compounds: sensory cues for health and nutritional value? *Science*, 311:815-819.

assumption in the pharmaceutical industry (and regulatory agencies) that negative side effects can be detected within that short testing period.

Health supplements are typically materials or extracts from plants that contain particular compounds that are perceived to have a beneficial effect on human physiology. They are bioactive molecules that affect animal physiology in some way. Most plants have dozens to hundreds of them. Examples are caffeine, nicotine, and morphine. These compounds are typically in relatively low doses in the plants because, let's remember, these compounds (i.e., secondary metabolites) in plants are toxins produced by the plant to kill or ward off herbivores, usually small insects.

The majority of medicines existing today are derived from or inspired by these plant toxins. Pharmaceutical companies employ chemists to identify and extract the bio-active compounds from plants, purify them, magnify the dose, and then design a delivery system that can be tolerated by humans. It is important to note that the process is one of isolating the active molecule *from its natural context*, which eliminates possible important interactions with other compounds in the plant. However, this is done because pharmaceutical effectiveness is based on a testing procedure that demands a rapid response and demonstrable effects of a single variable. Plant extracts cannot be tested in this way and rarely meet the criteria for being "effective."

However, by eating a plant-based diet, we get small doses of a large number of bioactive compounds every time we eat. If a certain plant is a normal part of the human diet and we are exposed to it regularly over long periods of time, we are receiving a low dose of a potentially medicinal stimulus from that plant every time we eat it. That stimulus could be from a single compound, from several compounds, or from interactions among the compounds. Almost certainly, the stimulus will be subtle and the benefits will be expressed slowly.

If the Mediterranean cuisine or Indian cuisine or other ethnic food palettes are considered intrinsically healthy, it is because of the characteristic plants and plant-derived seasonings that comprise those foods. Every meal contains low doses of medicinal chemicals in which people of those cultures are immersed over the course of their lives.

Is food medicine? Yes. Can plant-based supplements be medicine? Yes. If you take supplements for an extended period of time, it is certainly possible there will be subtle and even large positive effects. It is also possible that if you were not raised from childhood on foods containing those compounds, the effectiveness might be different from those who were raised on that diet.

What we can say is this: a long-term diet that is based on a variety of strongly flavored plants and plant seasonings is probably providing a medicinal boost to the human body. Plants are food for the microbiome and the microbiome is part of the foundation of our immune system. Secondary compounds in plants taken in small amounts may influence the diversity and functioning of the microbiome and thereby have indirect effects on human health. But it doesn't happen overnight and the testing methodology of modern medicine is incapable of detecting it.

Therefore, if we assume that humans have possessed a microbiome for a million years, and the microbiome contains large numbers of mutualistic species, and plant materials are the food for the microbiome, then a diet that provides our microbiome with a variety of plants and plant compounds will be heathier for us than a diet without such variety.

Chapter 30

The Care And Feeding Of Your Microbiome

A number of fad diets have emerged in recent years that support microbiome health to some degree. These diets insist on whole, fresh, and unprocessed foods. They are usually centered on plants, but if not, they still focus on food quality. In general, fad diets are well-intentioned and are often philosophically focused on the health of the human as well as the health of the environment. None of them are specifically focused on the microbiome in the sense that we have discussed it here, but that understanding is creeping in. I'll go over some of the more popular diet options, but this is meant to be a comparison of diet approaches rather than a comprehensive discussion of the merits of fad diets.

Obviously, any vegan, vegetarian, and macrobiotic diet will support the microbiome most directly. These mostly or wholly plant-based diets are challenging for many people because of the perception that they lack sufficient PFC components (protein, fat, carb) to meet our metabolic needs. That perception is rooted in the belief that the plant-based diet is made up primarily of the leafy parts of plants, which are low in oils, starch, and protein, but high in fiber and micronutrients.

While this viewpoint is true of the "vegetable" parts of the plant, the fruits, seeds, and roots tend to contain high levels of one or more of the high-calorie components and also have many important micronutrients. The perception that a plant-based diet lacks sufficient protein for maintaining muscle mass ignores the many high-energy and high-protein food options that are part of the plant-based diet. So, let's consider the basics of a few of the (currently) popular diet plans and how well they support both the microbiome and metabolic (caloric) needs.

Diets emphasizing unprocessed foods, such as the Raw or Paleo diets, are supportive of the microbiome. These diets are plant-based and the focus is to eliminate processed foods and other modern manipulations that reduce the natural nutrients of the food. Following a raw food diet is tricky because of the orientation of modern culture to highly cooked and processed foods. One of the important considerations is including enough PFC calories, but this is not a significant problem because fruits, seeds, and roots complement green vegetables, and meat can be included in the diet.

The Paleo diet has perhaps a stronger focus on seeds and fruits that can have a high protein content and often a high-fat content, and meat is a popular component. From the microbiome perspective, it is important to remember that plants should be a primary focus and, from a historical perspective, hunter and gatherer cultures were highly dependent on plant materials. For most hunter and gatherer societies, hunting for meat was a constant activity, but plants formed the base of the diet.

These "pre-historical" diets are a conscious move away from modern processed foods and toward a diet that strongly supports the microbiome. Any of these diets that maintain a high level of fresh or unprocessed plant materials on a daily basis should promote microbiome health, diversity, and stability.

Diets emphasizing seasonal foods are also supportive of the microbiome. The Macrobiotic, Ayurvedic, and Seasonal diets recommend eating foods, mostly plants, grown in the current season and usually from local sources. On these diets, summer foods should be eaten in the summer and winter foods in winter. Of course, this greatly restricts the diversity of plant types in the diet to particular times of the year, and one's recipe box has to be adjusted accordingly.

One assumption of these diets is that the summer or winter metabolism of the human body may be better supported by food produced during that time of year. For example, humans may experience seasonal changes in our physiology that affect body fat deposition, hormonal patterns, and energy expenditure. We certainly see such changes in behavior and metabolism in many species of animals (and all plants). However, we know nothing at all about whether the composition of the microbiome is sensitive to changes in the external environment or whether the microbiome reflects changes in the human body as it adjusts to the external environment.

What we do know is that our modern life no longer requires us to shift our eating patterns because of food availability, and we can suspect this may influence the benefits we derive from the microbiome. For many people, an important consideration for an invariable diet that disregards seasons is that eating summer foods in winter requires those foods to be grown in distant places. Those foods are grown in other parts of the world, transported across thousands of miles, and require enormous amounts of energy by the time they get to market. This is not an environmentally sustainable practice, of course, but it also means the foods have been in storage for weeks to months and will not be as fresh.

Similar to seasonal diets, another approach is what we could term a *terroir diet*, that is, a diet based on the location where the foods are grown, which is also influenced by the season. Such diets would include Mediterranean, Indian, Nordic, and Locavore diets that emphasize the influence of location on the quality of the foods.

This emphasis implies that the plants we eat are conditioned by the local environment, especially the soil, and the qualities imbued in locally-grown plants are important for supporting the health of the people living in those localities. This philosophy extends to the animals that feed on those plants that are then eaten by humans.

The climate shapes the soils of every region. The rain and temperatures determine the kinds of plants that will grow and the ranges of adaptations the plants will have. The plants determine the diversity and abundance of all local animal species, including microbes. The chemical compounds plants produce to protect themselves from insects and microbes are all adaptations to the specific location. We can assume that humans living and eating in every environment are awash in the chemicals contained in the local plants and these plants have a conditioning effect on the microbiome.

From a microbiome perspective, all of these dietary approaches toward plant-based nutrition will provide support for the diversity and health of the bacterial community in the gut. These plant-based diets have one important commonality: a focus on fresh and non-processed plant materials. We don't know much about the movement of bacteria from the environment into the gut, but we know it is taking place. Eating raw, fresh, or unprocessed plants will increase the likelihood of consuming bacteria that are best at breaking down those particular plants. This movement of bacteria into the gut with the plant materials is the movement of environmental and genetic information into our body.

The flow of information into the gut will keep the microbiome flexible and up-to-date with regard to the world around us. Eating plants that have been highly processed, overcooked, or grown under unnatural conditions will lack many or all of those benefits. This should be particularly concerning to everyone because the vast majority of whole plant foods we buy at the supermarket are produced under conditions that are designed to reduce and even eliminate the natural ecosystem.

Other popular diet plans tend to focus on "good and bad" in terms of PFC food types. While programs like Weight Watchers have no penalty for plants, the emphasis of the diet is to get participants to recognize "problem" foods and, not surprisingly, those are exclusively PFC foods. Many fad diets tend to support the microbiome (well, more so than in the past), but all have restrictions based on perceived negative aspects of certain foods, including some plants. In other words, a great many fad diets are exclusively concerned with metabolic foods – those that provide calories for the body – and less on foods that feed the microbiome.

The majority fit into the "low-carb" fad diets for which certain types of plants are restricted, such as sweet fruits and roots. (e.g., Atkins, South Beach, Keto, Paleo). These diets avoid high glycemic index sugars (Atkins and South Beach) and "modern" carb-rich plants (Paleo) or just carbs altogether (Keto). However, the "high protein" fad diets typically focus on meat, dairy, and plant-extract-based protein such as tofu. Plants are "allowed," but the emphasis is often a one-size-fits-all approach when it comes to carbs (which is more or less true of all recent fad diets). That is, *these diets tend to consider carb calories as "bad calories"* regardless of their origin.

As most dieters are focused first on weight loss and second on overall health, it might be worth noting that plant-based diet plans, especially those focused on unprocessed foods, are almost impossible to gain weight on. Indeed, it would be a challenge to eat a diet based exclusively on oil-rich whole plant foods such as seeds, nuts, and legumes and manage to gain weight. And the more of each plant (i.e., leaves and stems) that is included in the diet, the harder that would be. Regardless of the caloric content, the more one focuses on following a diet with the health of the microbiome in mind, the easier it is to forget about calories.

A plant-based diet is self-limiting in the sense that it's hard to overeat. Consider this: If I make mashed potatoes with four large potatoes, I could probably eat most of it (seriously, I could.). However, I can eat only one whole baked potato, and even then, I might not be able to eat the rest of my dinner. I can eat a large jar of apple sauce, but I can only eat one whole apple. Why? Because when I'm eating only a part of a food, my stomach does not receive or send the same signals about being full as when I'm eating the whole food. Foods that are derived from parts of plants (for example, processed foods) do not generate the same sensations of "satiety," and overeating is easy. In addition, processed foods are quick to digest, contain more easy-to-digest calories, and the feeling of satiety is short-lived.

And so, whether we follow a personal diet plan, a commercial diet program, or just follow our nutritional wisdom (i.e., our gut), *our focus should be on a diet that emphasizes plants that are as fresh and whole as possible.* Eat as much green vegetables and whole fruits as you want. Eat the whole fruit and vegetable whenever possible. Eat them raw or lightly cooked. Eat as great a diversity of plants as you can, and that includes seeds and nuts. Don't worry about plant fats. Eat strongly flavored plants and use plant-based seasonings.

The bottom line? Assume that expressing your full potential as a human will require all 400 secondary compounds found in the garden tomato and not just the 30 associated with the "tomato" flavor in the greenhouse tomato.

Listen to your body. As you get more and more in tune with your diet, you will find yourself craving or desiring certain flavors and foods. By this, I don't mean craving PFC-based foods and an urge to binge on ice cream. I'm referring to a desire for certain herbs or flavors or fruits. When eating food makes you feel better, it may well be food you need. When eating food results in a good feeling, we tend to gravitate to that food again. This "good feeling" may be related to the nutrients contained in that food, and that craving may be a hint that your body needs more of those nutrients. This is what is meant by "nutritional wisdom." However, be aware of the desire for foods (such as highly engineered fast foods and junk foods) that prey on our deep-seated attraction to sugar or salt. You can't hear the quiet inner voice of food wisdom over the clamor created by highly addictive components in junk foods.

Remember who you are eating for. The microbiome gets only leftovers. If food can be easily digested and absorbed in the 90-minute race through the convolutions of the small intestine, it will not reach the colon. Tougher materials that can't be broken down in that amount of time will make it to the slow, warm, anaerobic confines of the large intestine. The slow march through the much-shorter and wider colon is ten times longer than the small intestine. This is the time needed for bacteria to attack and decompose the tough cellulose molecules that make up plant fiber. You eat for the microbiome when you eat slow food.

What about meat? Eating meat is an ethical and moral decision that everyone has to make. I have some additional comments about meat production when I discuss the modern system of producing meat. However, meats are PFC and are for you as an individual, not for you as an ecosystem. All processed grains are for you as an individual. All fried food. All baked goods. And it's probably not surprising that just about anything you are tempted to binge on is a processed PFC food. If it comes in a box at the store, that food is for you, not for your microbiome. Consider it carefully because it has been designed by the food industry to generate a craving that is based on largely empty but abundant calories.

Occasional processed foods will not kill you. Like plant toxins, they are not inherently bad in small amounts. If your diet is plant-centered, eating a donut once in a while may be a pleasure. The PFC foods are not poison if the diet is oriented around maintaining a healthy microbiome. It's not cheating to eat pizza, but whole vegetables come first and more frequently. Having said that, the world of modern, highly processed, engineered-for-taste, fast food and junk food is not a healthy place for a dynamic and vibrant ecosystem like your microbiome. These foods are designed to be attractive to your head, not to your gut, and they are insidiously addictive. We grew up with these foods and they are hard to resist.

Something to keep in mind, however, is this: most foods, whether whole or processed, have probably decreased in quality over the past couple of decades. You may try to start dinner with a familiar healthy salad, but that salad has changed its character over the past few decades because of the methods and technology we now use to grow crop plants.

In fact, the loss of food quality is a slow process that has been happening in every facet of food production, whether processed or unprocessed. This is a serious problem if we are trying to increase the percentage of healthy foods in our diet yet relying on a commercial food production system that does not inherently value the qualities we are looking for in that food. This is now where we find ourselves, and this is the topic of the next chapter.

Chapter 31

What Is Food Quality?

"Nevertheless, there is a substantial and growing body of evidence to support the claim that nutrient content of intensively bred crops has dropped as yield has increased and time to harvest has decreased. Modern cultivars have been continuously selected for rapid growth and yield and, for the most part, have not been selected or even screened for nutrient content."[81]

There is one last item to consider regarding a high-quality diet based on plants that support our microbiome, and that is the problem of finding high-quality plants. This problem has become perhaps my greatest concern. It does us little good to eat lots of plants if the plants are of low quality and, unfortunately, the products we're being offered in the grocery store are on a rapid decline in that regard.

To be clear, I consider plant quality to be a measure of two things: *cellulose* and *secondary compounds*. Both of these, in turn, are products of a plant expressing its full genetic potential, and that expression is *only likely to occur under normal growing conditions and given a sufficient amount of time*. We have come full circle to the introduction of this book, where I used the tomato as an example to express this point. However, the loss of quality applies to almost all foods that we currently eat.

Concerns about food quality have grown as the food production system has become ever more dependent on chemicals, pesticides, fertilizers, genetic modification, and advanced technology for enhancing growth and production. The number of books making

---

[81] H.J. Klee and D.M. Tieman. 2013. Genetic challenges of flavor improvement in tomato. *Trends in Genetics*, 29:257-262.

claims about food and food production in relation to our health and the health of the surrounding ecosystem is hard to keep up with.[82]

The loss of genetic variation in crop plants that leads to a loss in food quality has been a talking point since the 1950s; Reginald Painter at Kansas State University was among the first to suggest that the emphasis on breeding for particular strains of our crops was the wrong direction to take. His primary point was this: in crop fields where there was more genetic variation, the losses to insect pests were lower. He was concerned that breeding for crop uniformity and, therefore, for low genetic variation would lead to a loss of resistance and a greater reliance on pesticides. In his view, we should focus research on maintaining genetic variation and understanding how that could be used to produce more robust crops.

Instead of heeding Painter's advice, the agricultural research world went rapidly in the opposite direction to focus on breeding for higher productivity, faster growth, more uniformity, and a predictably higher, *much higher*, reliance on technology. The loss of genetic potential in crops has reduced the capacity of those plants to express the full range of secondary compounds that are part of the species' heritage. As a consequence, our plant foods are slowly losing their nutritional value.

Like a snowball rolling down a hill, agricultural technology was increasingly geared toward producing strains of crops with hugely increased productivity and much faster growth. Today, we marvel not only at the levels of productivity but also at the ingenious technological strategies for eliciting that productivity from the crops. Initially, the increase was due to artificial fertilizers, then to breeding programs for faster growing plants, but now an entire industry is devoted to manipulating the genetics of crops to grow indoors, without soil, with uniform taste and texture and predictability.

As consumers, we think nothing of this process because we have come to believe that we will always have technology to solve our food problems. But what if this IS the source of declining food quality? What if, as Klee and Tieman say at the top of this chapter, this kind of food is not as good as it used to be? What are the repercussions to our health?

---

[82] Examples: *Insect resistance in crop plants* (Reginald Painter, 1951, Kansas Sate); *Chasing the Red Queen* (Andy Dyer, 2014, Island Press); *Food, Genes, and Culture* (Gary Paul Nabhan, 2013, Island Press); *The Omnivore's Dilemma* (Michael Pollan, 2006, Penguin); *Diet for a Dead Planet* (Christopher Cook, 2006, The New Press).

When plants are grown under artificial or highly modified conditions, what happens to them? For starters, plants grown quickly put little cellulose into their tissues. The leaves are soft and do not have the toughness needed to survive in the outside world. This physical reinforcement by cellulose occurs outdoors when the wind blows and the plants are forced to resist the wind.

When we buy pretty greenhouse plants, like small trees, for our yard that have been living a life of luxury in a protected environment with unlimited resources, they must be staked up, or the wind will blow them over. After a year or so of living outside, the plants can manage for themselves because the feedback from the environment has caused them to invest more in strong stems. UV radiation from the sun will cause leaves to become sturdier as well. The leaves of greenhouse plants often burn when planted in full sun because they are so weak and unprotected. When planted outdoors, those leaves will be replaced with newer, tougher leaves.

Plants living outside the greenhouse are forced to invest more in important structural parts, such as roots, stems, and leaves, whereas that investment was not necessary for growing in an environment that was shielded from nature. Unfortunately, greenhouse businesses that grow peppers and tomatoes are not interested in roots, stems, and leaves; they want fruit. Growers are not interested in plants that divert energy to stems when that energy could be diverted to making more fruit.[83] And so, the crop breeders produce strains of peppers and tomatoes that divert energy to fruit and less energy to strong, rigid stems. And they have produced plants that can tolerate, perhaps even require, the greenhouse environment.

In modern greenhouse and hothouse operations, there is little to no actual soil. If any soil is used, it is more or less sterile in the sense that normal bacteria, fungi, and nematodes are not present. Actual inorganic components such as sand, silt, and clay are not present either; the soil is an artificial "growth medium." All nutrients are delivered to the plant in the irrigation water, as are most of the systemic pesticides. The air around the plants moves at a constant speed because of electric fans; heaters and coolers are used to maintain optimal and uniform temperatures. Light intensity is adjusted with

---

[83] A recent and alarming discovery for me was being introduced to modern apple farming. Today more and more apples are being grown not on trees, but on (essentially) vertical poles with no branches. The ideal tree is about two feet wide and ten feet tall and can be harvested mechanically.

artificial lights, and any sunlight is indirect because of the indoor conditions.

In the greenhouse, no insects are desired unless bees, for example, are brought in specifically for pollinating flowers. Chemical use is frequent, if not constant, because of the threat of invasive pests such as aphids, whiteflies, spider mites, and a number of other tiny nuisances. And the plants grow extraordinarily fast and large because not only is less energy being diverted to structure (the plants are physically supported), the plants divert little to no energy to defend against insects. The conditions are ideal, the stresses are minimized, and the plants are factory-style production units. This is how you get a modern tomato.

This approach to food production can be applied to any annual plant and some perennial plants. In the produce section of literally all major grocery stores, you will find strawberries, blackberries, tomatoes, melons, zucchini, cucumbers, broccoli, celery, parsley, herbs, and many more, and at any time of year. Depending on where you live in this world, all or nearly all of these plants may have been grown indoors.

With the application of high-tech equipment, it just isn't cost-effective to grow these kinds of foods in uncontrolled outdoor environments where the watering, feeding, trimming, and harvesting processes are not completely uniform, and the losses to pests and weather can be highly unpredictable. Farms that are trying to produce food in the old-fashioned way are quickly going out of business unless they can market their produce through local stores, farmer's markets, or restaurants. But even so, they will be producing and selling a fraction of the quantity of the commercial, factory-style systems.

The result of an emphasis on productivity and speed is physically weak plants that disperse all available energy among a much larger number of fruits than is normal for the type of plant. Those fruits are often harvested well before they are truly ripe and before the plant has an opportunity (if it even possesses the ability) to invest in secondary chemicals, such as defense compounds, antioxidants, flavors, and vitamins that give the fruit its natural qualities.

Obviously, taste is one of those desirable qualities of our crop plants, but taste is derived from the mixture of the many chemicals the plants produce, many of which occur late in the ripening process, and many of those are why we enjoy eating the particular plant. That is, the subtle health benefits of *plants as slow medicine* are found in the complete plant, not the strange, inbred, genetically incomplete plant that now adorns the shelves of the produce section at the grocery store.

The quality is being bred out of the plants, and we should care. We are what we eat, and we want to eat real food because our microbiome is also what we eat, and it needs real tomatoes.

If establishing a diverse microbiome at birth is important, then no less important is maintaining that diversity for the rest of one's life. This maintenance can only be done through the consumption of diverse foods containing slow-to-digest materials, and most of this comes from unprocessed, outdoor-grown plants. A major component of shepherding a diverse microbiome as one ages is being able to avoid or recover from events, such as antibiotics, that damage the microbiome.

Unfortunately, coincident with the development of antibiotics after 1945 has been the inexorable development and adoption of a modern diet, usually called The Western Diet. We can also call this the PFC Diet: high in carbs, fats, sugars, and processed grains, low in fiber content, and in which fresh fruits and vegetables are a small percentage of the total.

The diet of Americans, for example, has gained 500 calories in the past few decades just from sugary drinks, and this was a result of the development of high fructose corn syrup. A technological breakthrough in 1980 created a rapid and inexpensive way to produce corn syrup, and immediately the cost of sweeteners for many different foods and drinks dropped dramatically. Selling sugary drinks became a huge moneymaker in the US and around the world because syrups were no longer the limiting factor in sodas. And we began to consume huge amounts of what my mother called "empty calories"; that is, calories that did nothing to reduce my youthful appetite but which I found delightful. An increase of 500 calories per day over basal metabolic needs equates to a weight gain of about one pound per week.[84]

---

[84] FOOD MATH: One pound equals 16 ounces, an ounce equals 28.3 grams, and there are 9 calories per gram of fat. Thus, one pound of fat equals ~4000 calories. To lose one pound of fat, one must burn about 4000 calories over and above what one consumes. If the standard diet is 2000 calories per day, one could try not eating for two days to lose a pound or one could reduce food intact by 500 calories for a week. Unless one is over-weight by hundreds of pounds, losing weight fast is not easy (or healthy), and losing weight slowly is frustrating and requires determination. To begin, however, if a person stopped consuming empty calories, such as the 500 sugar calories the average American drinks each day, losing a pound a week could be possible without even exercising.

It is weird to think that the combination of an ever-lower quality diet and the frequent use of antibiotics has forced us to think of the maintenance of a healthy microbiome as an intentional act instead of a natural process. Historically, we never had to wonder if the food we were eating was good for us and now *everything* at the store requires scrutiny of the nutritional contents by the conscientious consumer. Of course, we have to worry that anything new might actually be bad for us, but is it right that we have to be concerned about foods that have always been the definition of "good food"?

Chapter 32

How Fast Should Our Food Be?

Fast Industrial Plants

So, here we are. All plants are like tomatoes. For the full expression of their genetic potential, they need to live in healthy soil, experience wind and rain and heat, and fend off hungry insects. They need to be challenged by their environment in ways that cause them to express their adaptations for survival. For that to happen, they need to grow at a natural rate of development with adequate time spent in each phase of life. The negative interactions with the living and non-living environment temper the plants and make them stronger and tastier. Ultimately, the production of each plant is limited by the amount of energy it can capture from the sun (or overhead rack of lights), and this light energy has to be distributed amongst the many different parts of the plant that require energy for growing. Basically, that's the starting point for understanding plants.

The push for higher productivity in modern agriculture is an attempt to take the finite amount of energy a plant has but divide it among a greater number of products. And one result is lower quality products. As an example of why this decrease in quality occurs, consider a peach tree that is large enough to produce enough energy for 100 large fruits. The energy is finite because the tree has a certain surface area of leaves and they can intercept only a certain amount of sunlight. If I force that same plant to produce 200 fruits, the available energy for each fruit will be half of what it was. And if I force the plant to produce those fruits in half the time, each fruit will have less than ¼ of its original energy because the plant has less time to collect that energy. The result is less sugar and fewer secondary compounds, less flavor, and lower nutritional quality.

If we breed the plant to produce fruits that are the same size as before, each fruit will have higher water content and will seem less sweet. This works great if I'm a seller and I sell by the pound, but not so great if I'm a consumer. Previously, where I might eat, let's say, one peach to get my daily dose of Vitamin C, now I have to eat four or more peaches for the same level of nutrition. One potential consequence is that we, the consumers, can be undernourished by eating food that no longer delivers the goods.

Even worse, if we listen to the nutritional wisdom of our bodies, we may be hearing a message to compensate for that lack of nutrition by eating more, and that will result in overeating.[85] Additionally, and importantly, the lower density of cellulosic compounds in this factory-style production system of weak, young plant products is essentially starving our microbiome and making us feel hungry more often.

Modern technology and the rising demand for food by a growing human population have pushed agriculture in this direction. The intentions of plant scientists have always had an altruistic impetus: to find ways to feed a hungry world efficiently. The commercial side of the agricultural industry, of course, is largely driven by the profit motive, and the goals, especially since the 1950s, have focused on speed, production, and marketability.

These dual goals of producing more food and making greater profits have resulted in industrial uniformity, which is also a result of reduced genetic variation and of intense breeding for rapid and predictable production by crop plants. The result has been a slow but perceptible diminution of *food quality*. We don't see it on a day-to-day basis, but ask anyone over the age of 50 whether the foods they ate as a child taste the same as today.

For efficient commercial production, these changes are considered positives and, of course, marketing strategies will always focus on the positives. For example, if children are more likely to eat bland vegetables, then bland vegetables will sell better than the alternatives. Sweet corn now has a 12% higher sugar content and much less "corn" flavor compared to 30-40 years ago. We used to eat spinach that took several weeks to grow, but now we are being convinced to buy "baby spinach," which is the small leaves from

---

[85] While vitamin supplements are largely unnecessary when one eats a healthy plant-based diet, if our modern plants are, in fact, depleted or diluted in nutrient contact, it may be necessary to supplement our diet with vitamins and minerals to some extent. This has yet to be decided or even investigated (to my knowledge).

spinach that can be produced in just days under factory greenhouse conditions. Baby spinach is easier to chew and doesn't have that slightly bitter spinach flavor. Romaine lettuce used to be a "tastier" alternative to the flavor-free Iceberg lettuce, but today Romaine is grown so rapidly it is indistinguishable from its tasteless cousin.

And, as the fast-food industry has discovered and encouraged, food does not have to be inherently tasty; flavors can be added and public opinion can be manipulated. If you pay attention to advertisements for food, particularly in the fast-food market, you may have noticed that the focus is entirely on the added flavors rather than the natural flavors.

For ourselves, *we have to recognize that food quality is found in natural flavors*. Those flavors tell us about the qualities of the plant. The presence of those flavors tells us the plant grew slowly, overcame environmental stress, and had the opportunity to mature before it was harvested. Thus, the quality of the plant can be found in the aging process, much like the qualities that slowly emerge in a good red wine. These products of aging are not the PFC foods that energize our physical bodies. Rather, they are the food supply for our microbiome and they are the slow medicines we have evolved with and expect from our food. For those of us who want to eat high-quality plant material to feed our microbiome, our desires are at odds with modern food production methods, which are focused on speed and efficiency. *Speed is the enemy of quality,* and this is especially true for growing high-quality plants for food.

Fast Industrial Meat

Animals are not plants, but when it comes to quality, there can be some important parallels. In this regard, we have done unto animals raised for meat as we have done unto plants. As other authors have described in detail,[86] the meat we eat today is made from corn, is raised and harvested as quickly as possible, is removed from the natural environment to the greatest degree possible, and is completely dependent on chemical and medical technology. While our microbiome does not in any way depend on meat, the health of our microbiome depends on the health of our environment, and meat production is part of that environment. For humans out there who

---

[86] Examples: *Food Inc: A Participant Guide* (Karl Weber, 2009, PublicAffairs); *Big Chicken* (Maryn McKenna, 2017, National Geographic); *CAFO: The Tragedy of Industrial Animal Factories* (Daniel Imhoff, 2010, Earth Aware).

consider themselves carnivores, the quality of the meat-production environment should be of great concern.

The beef we eat is mostly year-old old steers who spent the last three months of their lives eating nothing but corn-based feed (with antibiotics and additives) to gain 100 pounds a month, a great deal of which is fat. The flavor of cooked beef today is largely due to the searing of fat. The standard five-pound chicken at the store was raised on corn-based feed (plus antibiotics) in just about a month and a half. The flavor of modern chicken is added by breading or flavoring. Pigs? Yes, fed corn and corn byproducts. Farm-raised salmon? Yes, now raised on corn.[87]

True grass-fed free-range beef does not taste the same as corn-fed feedlot beef. Free-range chickens have flavors that cannot be found in a commercially produced chicken. In fact, "dark" meat and "white" meat are not easy to distinguish anymore because the commercial chicken is incapable of using the running muscles in its legs. A wild salmon spends two years in the ocean before returning to its freshwater birthplace. That's two years of survival, feeding on wild foods, and that experience adds true seasoning to its muscles. Free-range meats are leaner and have a stronger, gamier flavor. These are characteristics that will not be found in factory-style meat production because, again, the qualities of the organism depend on the challenges faced in the environment. A war veteran has real stories to tell; a couch potato only has imaginary stories.

And animals are what they eat. Today, we eat animals that have been fed a uniform diet and are nearly uniform in flavor. That is, they are uniformly tasteless and ready for flavor to be added. While the microbiome may not depend on the proteins and fats from meat, there are other qualities to wild food that we do not understand well. We may not depend on our meat for nutrients other than protein and fats, but we have absolutely no idea how the cholesterol and other chemicals in those meats interact with our system. We have no idea whether animals raised on antibiotics can transfer unknown residual effects to the eater of the meat.

However, we do know that cow's milk from cows raised on growth hormones can have unintended effects on a child's

---

[87] If meat, eggs, or dairy products are labeled with some reference to increased Omega-3 fatty acids, it is likely the corn diet of the animal was enhanced with flaxseed. However, Omega-3 content will also be higher in dairy products from grass-fed cows.

development. That by itself should be a reason to reconsider all other chemicals that are applied to the food we eventually eat, and that would include the plants the animals eat. Nonetheless, if we believe that plants contain chemicals with medicinal qualities and those compounds are lost in the modern farm system, then we should also be concerned that other kinds of food that are treated similarly, such as meats, may be missing important qualities as well.

Chapter 33

Take Control Of Your Diet (And Your Microbiome)

The food and flavor industries have taken over the job of adding taste to our food[88]. And we are being encouraged to accept that decision and that process. With every petition to the Food and Drug Administration to market genetically modified, genetically uniform, highly inbred crops that produce food items that are easy to harvest, pick, pack, ship, store, cook, eat, and are pretty to look at, we are losing quality in our foods.

And while the food industry has convinced the FDA that there are no "significant" differences between the old crops and the new crops, we are ceding control of our diet to grossly uninformed and commercial-based decision making. Our diet is the basis of our health, and our food is being produced with commercial profit in mind, not consumer health. We not only have simplified the environment, but we have allowed the crops we want to grow in the environment to be simplified. The result is food that does not support the things that require complexity. Those things, of course, would be us as individuals and, more importantly, our internal ecosystem.

In this regard, Aldo Leopold (from *Round River*, 1972) should be a source of guidance.

"The last word in ignorance is the man who says of an animal or plant, "What good is it?" If the...whole is good, then every part is good, **whether we understand it or not***. If the biota, in the course of*

---

[88] Mark Schatzker. 2015. *The Dorito Effect*. Simon and Schuster.

aeons, has built something we like but do not understand, then who but a fool would discard seemingly useless parts?" (Emphasis added)

If the food we make does not support our microbiome, which is the source of our physiological flexibility, our defense system, and our capacity to respond to changes in our environment, then this action is equivalent to us discarding 99% of our available genes. On top of that, our environment is definitely changing. At no point in our history has this been more evident.

We have become so disconnected from the source of our health (especially from the production of food) that we are actually confused about what we should be eating to be healthy, which is both amazing and tremendously alarming. We cannot depend on the food industry to educate us on that point because it is the food industry, from farming to processing, that has been leading the charge to keep food prices low at the expense of food quality. This process has been continuous and accelerating since the 1950s and is now the norm rather than a recent aberrancy. While we may appreciate the continued low cost of food, we are assuming the quality has not changed over time, and we are ignoring the basic rules of ecology, physics, chemistry, and even economics.

Today, our food, which is our source of nutrition and the slow medicine we take every day to stay healthy, is less and less a source of nutrition or slow medicine. As we assault our bodies with the constant barrage of chemicals that characterize human civilization in the 21st Century, we are being stripped of our natural protections. Our relationship with our environment is broken, and our bodies are not capable of defending us against an ever-changing world. There is little evidence that anything significant is being done to address this situation at a governmental level. Our legal protections related to food are focused on safety issues related to toxins (such as food dyes and pesticides), carcinogens (mostly additives), and allergens (certain food components).

In the US, there are no particular rules about food quality *per se* and very few laws protecting consumers against what *might be* dangerous. By that, I mean we are not protected against changes to foods that might affect food quality in ways that we can't yet predict or understand. Typically, discoveries about negative effects are made well after the fact, and institutional changes are only made grudgingly (and usually in response to litigation) and only after a great deal of data has been collected for many years.

And so, we must take control of our own health and we do that by *intentionally* strengthening our relationship with our microbiome through a high-quality diet.

Basic Rules Of Eating (And Shopping)

We need some guidelines for evaluating our food, and those guidelines must be based on the principles of evolutionary biology and should include what we suspect might be true. By that, I mean we must err on the side of caution. We don't have conclusive data about the nuances of the microbiome and food quality in relation to our day-to-day health, but *we can't wait for that eventuality*. In fact, the health food and fad diet industries have always taken this approach, but not for the same reasons that we should. Unfortunately, capitalism has a way of blinding good intentions such that the terms "good" and "bad" become watchwords for consumers, but with a lot of variation in the intended meaning.

The primary word of guidance for us should be "quality." And we should be wary of anything that reduces *what we understand to be quality*. We may not always know what "quality" is specifically, but we know enough to err on the side of caution.

I'm going to suggest some guidelines for selecting foods that will more or less imply quality, support the microbiome, and direct the chooser toward better foods. This is by no means an exhaustive list and readers should feel free to add their personal touches to their buying choices.

*****Fresh is best***. Food should be as fresh as possible with little to no prior processing. Such food can be eaten in its original state. Ideally, the food has been rinsed only with water and not with chemicals. The rinsing process should be needed only to remove dirt and unnecessary debris, but not as a necessary precaution against potential toxins, such as pesticides. Foods such as fruits that are stored for months in refrigerators (during and after shipping) are less desirable than those arriving directly from the field. Fresh foods may be our best source of appropriate probiotics (new bacteria). The processing and sterilizing procedures of the commercial food industry will diminish this source.

*****Slow to digest***. Perhaps this should be the first guideline, but the goal in selecting quality food is to remember the difference between PFC foods and microbiome foods. PFC foods will tend to be more processed and will not resemble the original organism. That includes meats, which are increasingly treated before, during, and after processing with chemicals. Plants are prebiotics; the original compounds found in plants are the substances that feed the microbiome. Slow-to-digest foods also give a greater sense of satiety which assists in curbing the desire to eat again. *Use this criterion of satiety as a measure of your food quality.*

Feed your microbiome first. This is a corollary to the previous statement, but it's so important it should be said twice. As an individual, you need 1500-2000 calories a day to meet your metabolic needs. You'll get them, don't worry, but a focus on the microbiome implies a focus on food quality. Eating more plant material will reduce your PFC calorie intake because you will not feel as hungry after feeding the microbiome. I predict that as you focus on meeting the needs of the microbiome, you will have less desire to eat lower quality foods anyway. A healthy microbiome requires the highest quality plants you can consume, and remember that high quality, in this sense, means cellulose and secondary compounds. That is, *high-quality plants are chewy and naturally flavorful.*

Organic implies probiotic. Field-gown produce is more likely to possess probiotic bacteria if it is grown without pesticides. The bacteria associated with commercially grown produce will also be bacteria that can survive the chemical environment of the commercial farm. While this does not necessarily imply unhealthy, these are not the bacterial strains of the natural ecosystem and are likely to be bacteria that are resistant to chemical treatments. While we know little about the recruitment of new bacteria into our microbiomes, we know that there is flux and the new arrivals must be coming from our environment. And it makes sense that a healthy food production environment will be less likely to harbor harmful bacteria.

Consider your probiotic environment. As a follow-up to the previous guideline, research on the development of the microbiome in toddlers indicates a strong influence of family members and the people we live with later in life. That means *we are sharing our microbiomes* with our housemates. This should have a protective aspect because new bacteria increase our personal diversity. When a shared community (such as a household) experiences similar health problems, it does not necessarily mean a genetic predisposition because it can also mean an unhealthy probiotic environment. In other words, *we are what we eat, but it also may be true that we are what those around us eat.*

Challenge the microbiome. Expand your variety of plant foods. The greater the variety of foods, the greater the diversity of bacteria you are supporting in your colon. Diversity is the cure for many things. It prevents an unhealthy dominance by a small number of bacterial species. It can prevent gastric upset and flatulence after eating new and different foods. Ecological studies have shown that more diverse systems can extract a greater quantity and variety of resources from the environment. We can assume that a diverse microbiome is better able to provide a greater variety of nutrients than a depleted microbiome. *Exercise your digestive system with a diverse diet.*

Quality comes with age. Most of us want to hear that, but what I mean is this: Eat plants that are grown slower, take longer, have stronger flavors, and are chewier. (Unfortunately, they might also be more expensive.) These plants are not always the prettiest. Food producers are acutely aware of food appearance, and young foods are prettier because they haven't had the exposure to pests or the time to age. Yes, age can take its toll on appearance, but age implies maturity and, for plants, that maturity is the foundation of quality. *Skip the baby foods; go for foods with life experience.*

Superfoods are real. They're called plants. However, eating plant extracts is not the same as eating the actual plant. When medicines are developed from plants, the active chemical is isolated, purified, concentrated, and then packaged in a delivery system. Whatever context that chemical was in while part of the plant is lost. The slow medicines that are in plants are in their original context, which typically means in the presence of many other slow medicines. We do not understand the importance of the natural cocktail of these chemicals with regard to their actions as slow medicine. We may never untangle that knot, but we can trust that the context is important. *Eat the plant, not the extracts.*

Eat whole foods. Don't peel fruits or roots; always eat the skin. The skin (or peel or rind) usually has many nutrients not found in the sweet or starchy areas. And the skin is mostly cellulose. The skin (cellulose) is complex and provides information to your digestive system that helps reduce the sensation of hunger and thereby reduces overeating. While the juicing fad is a healthy fad, I would advocate for smoothies that incorporate whole foods rather than juicing, which saves the liquid but discards most of the cellulose. *Eat like an adult.*

Shop with an attitude. Try to be an environmentally, ecologically, and scientifically responsible consumer. It is hard to know how much genetic alteration and breeding our produce has been subjected to in order to get the marketable characteristics we see at the store. *Assume it's a lot*. We should understand that any plant that requires only a short time to grow is being manipulated and probably has been for decades. In part, this is because breeding efforts for short-lived plants can be conducted in months rather than years. On the other hand, tree fruits and nuts are less modified than the plants that can be grown indoors. That isn't to say they haven't been as subjected to breeding for improvements, but a tree typically requires several years of growing before it produces fruit or nuts, and that is a major investment for farmers. And as the perennial plant ages, it produces food with greater chemical complexity (to which everyone in the wine industry will attest.)

Learn your food sources. In addition to the above, find out where your fresh food was grown. Food produced in the US can travel 3000 miles to the market, will take days to get there, and is often picked at an unripe stage. Some fruits are treated with ethylene gas (a natural ripening hormone) to generate a "ripe" look by the time they get to their destination. On the other hand, grapes in winter and early spring come from Chile and Mexico, and bananas are from Central America. Ask other questions about your fresh food. Are there more local sources? Does the farmer have a human name and face? How was the food grown? For foods labeled "organic," meeting the letter of the law is not the same as meeting the intent of the law, and knowing something about the grower can be important. Some "all-natural" foods come from more responsible growers than do some "organic" foods. Educate yourself about the source of your food and how it was produced.

Question food longevity. Long shelf life implies missing ingredients, added ingredients, and always means preservatives. Products with a long shelf life are only distantly related to fresh foods. Long shelf life means the more volatile chemical components have been removed, and that often means vitamins and beneficial oils are missing. The extracted chemicals are then added back in a more stable form or left out. Personally, I have a concern about preservatives, even natural preservatives. If bacteria and fungi can't eat it, then should I? At issue is whether foods containing antimicrobial chemicals (i.e., preservatives) that can make it to the colon will have adverse effects on my beneficial bacteria. It is true that the secondary compounds produced by plants are often antimicrobial. But if we eat plants and we don't experience digestive distress, we are either breaking those compounds down ourselves, or our microbiome is coping with them. On the other hand, chemicals we add to food that suppress microbial growth are chemically stable (hence, long shelf life) and are not natural to our food environment, and I advise consumers to find out more about them or to avoid them.

I'm sure there are a number of other criteria we can use to assess the quality of our food. Indeed, you should probably make up a Quality Control Handbook for easy reference until you have your dietary guidelines firmly in your mind as you shop. However, the very act of asking questions about quality is an important starting point. It means you are taking control of your nutrition and, most importantly for this discussion, taking control of the health of your microbiome (and you as an ecosystem.)

If you would like a take-home message, it is this: **We need high-quality food to maintain a high-quality microbiome to support a healthy body**. Those foods are not PFC foods. However, our modern problems with diet are rooted not only in the production of low quality, mostly PFC foods, but also in the continued reduction in quality of our traditional non-PFC foods. We have to be smarter eaters. A healthy and diverse microbiome is likely to be the greatest tool we have for maintaining personal health, but only when the microbiome is supported by thoughtful and responsible eating behavior.

Epilogue

A World View Based On Quality

French winemakers understand the microbial world. They understand inherent complexity, particularly in the interactions between the grapevines and the land on which they grow. The results of those interactions are the grapes. French winemakers have given us a word for how the environment shapes the qualities of the grapes: *terroir* (pronounced ter-war).

Terroir is the influence of the thousands of different elements in the local environment on the organisms growing in that environment. The grapes are the vine's expression of its genotype living in that environment. The winemaker's job is to make wines that express the potential of the grapes.

The quality of the wine cannot be manufactured. Winemaking is a slow process of coaxing the terroir out of the grapes, and that terroir is expressed in the flavors and aromas of the countryside that became part of the grapes themselves. The grapevines live in that environment; they collaborate with and tolerate all of the plants and animals, they experience the seasons, they cycle with the soils, and the grapes produced each year reflect that life and that journey. *With the environment, the grape is the expression of potential; without the environment, the grape is just a fruit.*

Our health is also a product of our ecosystem and in much the same way. In a very real sense, *our complex omnivore digestive system is our superpower*. Because we are omnivores, we can sample nearly everything in the environment. In some ways, nothing is off-limits because the microbiome we carry with us provides the capacity for testing almost every plant for its potential as food. But we are at risk of losing that superpower, and we must work consciously and assiduously to maintain it. We must collaborate with our microbiome such that we allow it to express its potential relative to our human physiology. This mutualistic relationship is a slow dance, one that must be practiced and studied, and it does not happen overnight.

Terroir carries with it additional nuances. In vineyards, the terroir is derived from the soil type, the microbes in the soil, the slope and exposure of the hillside, and the seasonal changes affecting those factors. The plants, animals, and microbes interact with the soil and produce what ecologists call "legacy effects." That is, the lasting effects of the presence of those organisms even after they are gone. Thus, a soil that is damaged and depleted of microbes cannot provide the same complexity to the grapes as a stable, healthy, diverse soil. In other words, the quality of the grapes produced in a region depends on the health of the *other* organisms in that region, and the vines are not at their best unless the surrounding environment is intact and healthy.

And so it is with the expression of human potential, our "tomato-ness." Each of us relates to the environment in different ways. Each of us has our own particular microbiome, whether on the skin, in the mouth, or in the colon. Each of us has our personal history, and that determines how we react to stress. As a consequence, each of us will react differently as we each experience the same environmental stress. This is important.

The ability to react and the intensity of the reactions are modified by our prior experience. Our makeup, our capacity, is a function of the quality of the environment we have been living in. The more diverse and challenging the environment we have lived in previously, the more capable we are of handling new stressors now. Our external environment has given us that capacity by eliciting it from us. Every challenge we faced and overcame in the past has helped to condition and develop our ability to handle future challenges.

If our environment is impoverished, we will be impoverished. We will be handicapped in our ability to respond or to resist or to bounce back. We will be like greenhouse tomatoes lacking the qualities and characteristics that are inherent in our genetic makeup or in the makeup of our healthy microbiome. We will be like germ-free mice lacking a defense system that is absolutely a natural condition in a healthy being. And it is important to recognize that we depend on the internal ecosystem for our daily health, but we also depend on the external ecosystem for the stimuli that bring out our best and for the flow of information that maintains our internal ecosystem. Our microbiome is nested within us and we are nested within the ecosystem that surrounds us.

We know next to nothing about the details of the interactions between the human body and the microbiome and the infinite number of cascading effects those interactions likely influence. *But claiming a lack of knowledge is not an excuse for a lack of action.* Nobody has complete knowledge, and in the case of the microbiome, nobody has much of anything (despite what they might advertise to the contrary). We don't understand prebiotics, we don't understand probiotics, and we don't understand how our chemical world is affecting us internally. And that won't change much in the near future (despite what you might see in advertisements.). Our ignorance of the specifics matters, but it also doesn't matter.

If we understand that 30 trillion bacteria with 5 million genes in our internal ecosystem are working on our behalf by helping to maintain a healthy host and that we can help them by modifying our eating habits and by avoiding unnecessary anti-microbial dangers, then we have some degree of control over our own health.

If we recognize what a healthy external environment looks like, we have some measure of control over our own health. And we can take steps to improve one to improve the other.

Ultimately, given the road we are on with 8 billion people, mass-produced food, and life in megacities, we have little choice unless we resigning ourselves to a shortened life of poor health. To me, the choice is easy and the changes we can make in our lives are pretty easy too. And it is no more of a chore than shopping with my eyes open and paying attention.

Buy organic, buy natural, buy from local growers, shop the farmer's market, make food connections, create food co-ops, encourage local restaurants, read the labels, use your money to make a change, and use your voice to find other voices. Those who claim that high-quality foods are niche, or too expensive to make, or can't possibly feed the world, or aren't better for you are actually the Pollyannas of the world. They truly believe that life is great and all is well; food is cheap, food is flavorful, and all food is good for you. And that technology has and will continue to provide the answers. This is not about saying they're wrong. It's about recognizing that we are not alone and we have been ignoring our partners.

About The Author

I am a professor at the University of South Carolina Aiken (since 2000), where I teach botany, ecology and evolution, environmental science, restoration ecology, and research methods. I have degrees in zoology and wildlife biology (BA, MA, from California State University, Fresno) and plant ecology (PhD from the University of California, Davis). Later I spent two years working in the Negev Desert in Israel (for the University of Michigan). My research focus is plant ecology and evolutionary biology, but, in general, I study how disruptions to natural systems affect the integrity and functioning of those systems.

In *Chasing the Red Queen: The Evolutionary Race Between Agricultural Pests and Poisons* (2014, Island Press), I used basic concepts from ecology and evolutionary biology to explain how the process of food production in modern agriculture has changed, how it adheres less and less to natural biological principles, and how technological interventions with pesticides and genetic modification will ultimately fail. The goal of the book was to raise awareness of the hazards inherent in ignoring the rules of evolutionary biology when it comes to food production and health. Essentially, that is also the focus of this second book.

My goal in writing is to inform the general public about science, particularly the basic principles of evolutionary biology, and how science can be applied to understanding everyday life. I believe people want to know more about science, particularly with regard to their health and well-being. As a writer, I want to explain the important concepts in an understandable way, but it's more important to me that readers have enough understanding to actually make decisions on their own rather than depending on other people to make decisions. Most readers do not have the time or desire to get a PhD, so it's up to writers to provide that understanding.

Made in the USA
Columbia, SC
24 September 2022